AF834978

EMPOWERING CHILDREN TO COPE WITH DIFFICULTY AND BUILD MUSCLES FOR MENTAL HEALTH

EMPOWERING CHILDREN TO COPE WITH DIFFICULTY AND BUILD MUSCLES FOR MENTAL HEALTH

Eric L. Dlugokinski, Ph.D.
Sandra F. Allen, Ph.D.

Department of Psychiatry and Behavioral Sciences
The University of Oklahoma Health Sciences Center
Oklahoma City, Oklahoma

Routledge
Taylor & Francis Group
LONDON AND NEW YORK

EMPOWERING CHILDREN TO COPE WITH DIFFICULTY AND BUILD MUSCLES FOR MENTAL HEALTH

First published 1997 by Accelerated Development

Published 2018 by Routledge
2 Park Square, Milton Park, Abingdon, Oxon OX14 4RN
52 Vanderbilt Avenue, New York, NY 10017

First issued in hardback 2018

Routledge is an imprint of the Taylor & Francis Group, an informa business

Copyright © 1997 Taylor & Francis

All rights reserved. No part of this book may be reprinted or reproduced or utilised in any form or by any electronic, mechanical, or other means, now known or hereafter invented, including photocopying and recording, or in any information storage or retrieval system, without permission in writing from the publishers.

Notice:
Product or corporate names may be trademarks or registered trademarks, and are used only for identification and explanation without intent to infringe.

This book was set in Times Roman. The editor was Judith L. Aymond. Technical development by Cynthia Long. Cover design by Michelle Fleitz.

A CIP catalog record for this book is available from the British Library.

Library of Congress Cataloging-in Publication Data

Dlugokinski, Eric L.
Empowering children to cope with difficulty and build muscles for mental health/Eric L. Dlugokinski, Sandra F. Allen.
p. cm.
Includes bibliographical references and index.
1. Child mental health. 2. Children—Life skills guides. 3. Mental health—Study and teaching (Elementary) 4. Adjustment disorders in children—Prevention. 5. Adjustment (Psychology) in children. I. Allen, Sandra F. II. Title.
RJ499.D57 1996
618.92′89—dc20 96-35133
CIP

ISBN 13: 978-1-138-46266-3 (hbk)
ISBN 13: 978-1-56032-497-3 (pbk)

CONTENTS

LIST OF FIGURES

LIST OF EXERCISES

OUR VISION FOR EMPOWERING CHILDREN

Our society focuses energy on removing problems once they appear. All of our energy devoted to treating these problems will not prevent new problems from occurring. A story illustrates our need for new approaches:

Imagine a group of children who have fallen in a deep river.
They are in danger of drowning.

Ten of us are downstream
Rescuing the children as they float down the river.
All of us are very busy
But we just can't save all the children who have fallen in.

We decide to send two or three of us upstream.
Their job is to look for ways
To prevent children from falling in the river.

Maybe we could build a fence around the cliff . . .
Or build new paths for children . . .
Or recruit family to teach children to swim,
Or find elders to teach children to stay
away from the cliffs.

Our vision is to train professionals and volunteers to go upstream. Our mission is to reach out to children and families in our community with effective strategies to empower children.

PREFACE

The task of growing up in today's society is becoming increasingly complex and hazardous. If growing up is about the business of becoming a competent, productive, and socially contributing adult, there are land mines everywhere. During the growing up years, even our children's physical survival is in jeopardy. Childhood mortality in the United States resulting from violence is the highest of eight industrialized countries studied (Wilson-Brewer, Cohen, O'Donnell, & Goodman, 1991). These authors cite research that violence in our schools and communities is escalating and becoming a domain of status and power for children. The peak of this violence is seen in their estimate that every day 135,000 children bring guns to school. Perpetrators and victims are both casualties.

Violence, however, is only one of many "risk factors" that our children face in growing up. Boys and girls of today's society face increasing risks of alcohol and drug abuse, unwanted pregnancy, delinquency, truancy, emotional disorders, sexually transmitted diseases, and school failure (Dryfoos, 1990). Recent incidence and prevalence estimates indicate that 50% of American youth are at a moderate or high risk for a variety of serious problem behaviors (Consortium on the School Based Promotion of Social Competence, 1991).

When we view that a child's major resource for buffering these risks, the family, is also troubled, the magnitude of these risk factors is alarming. More children live in divorced or single parent households than ever before. Adult resources for providing children's protection through nurturing and guidance are stretched to the limit.

Traditional methods of mental health intervention are inadequate to meet the needs of these children. If we combined all of our counselors and therapists, we still would have the capacity to reach only about one to two percent of these children through individual psychotherapy and counseling (Lewis, Dlugokinski, Caputo, & Griffin, 1988). Furthermore, the most disturbed of our children only attend five sessions or fewer of outpatient therapy (Sowder, Burt, Rosenstein, & Milazzo-Sayre, 1980).

Although the editors and authors of this book practice individual therapy with children and families, we are painfully aware that we need skill building mental health services of a new kind and dimension if we are to reach these children. Our health care costs are already astronomical. We must find a way to reach more children with skills that can protect them from becoming dysfunctional or disordered.

As the word prevention itself suggests, we need to find modes of intervention that come *before* our children become casualties of the various risks they face. Pransky (1991) argued for the viability of prevention approaches, because most disorders are intertwined and connected. Delinquency, emotional problems, drug abuse, teen pregnancy, and welfare dependency co-occur. Thus, if we can find ways to interrupt or protect children from some of these problems, we are also likely to be addressing other problems as well.

It is time to take what we know about forming mentally healthy lives out in the open. Skill building for self-control, healthy relationships, and coping have been well-kept secrets behind the closed doors of clinical practice to a selected few patients. It is time to bring these skills to the classroom where we can educate children to grow up into competent adults.

We cannot stand still. There is a danger that we can become immobilized in the face of all of these problems or remain static in our approach to mental health service delivery.

Recent work in the area of protecting children is encouraging. Protective factors, such as developing coping skills and positive pro-social relationships between children, can build children's resiliency (Hancock, Gager, & Elias, 1993; Hawkins, Catalano, & Miller, 1992; Jessor, 1991). The solutions are not simple or quick. The evidence suggests we need to offer our services intensively if they are to make a difference. One-shot efforts and simple solutions just do not work. We also need to involve parents, teachers, mentors, and other volunteers so that children can model healthy behavior on a day-by-day basis.

The authors of this book have been active for many years in both traditional psychotherapy and in educating children in the classroom. We have attempted to synthesize some of our experiences with information from the literature that we hope will be useful for preventive interventions in the classroom. We have chosen to focus on the early elementary school years. We view these years as critical to building healthy relationship and coping patterns. Our goal is to help counselors and mental health professionals empower our children with resiliency to avoid the land mines and to develop emotionally healthy ways of living.

INTRODUCTION

The broad goal of this book is to support counselors, mental health educators, and professionals in prevention with the background information and practical suggestions they need to help children learn emotionally healthy ways of thinking, living, and relating. These professionals also may find sections of this material useful in training volunteers to assist them. The objective is to assist professionals in their understanding and practice by providing conceptual and practical tools that they can use to build a reserve of emotional strength in our children.

Many of these practical suggestions for developing mental health skills in children can be employed with groups of children or adapted to meet the needs of individual children. Although these exercises were designed for use in schools, they might be applicable in other community settings where children meet on a regular basis.

Some professionals want to better understand research about children and the issues they face so they can relate to them more effectively. Others may be interested in practical, step-by-step suggestions for intervening in children's lives. The information contained in this book provides insight for professionals in both of these areas, and it is grounded in sound mental health practices and research.

Children's mental health issues have become increasingly complex. An attempt has been made to describe these issues in clear, straightforward language in as few pages as possible by integrating information where applicable.

The book is organized in two sections. Each section includes a literature review, research findings in the area, and practical suggestions.

Section I, Coping Skills, primarily is focused on helping children deal with problem situations. The section begins with a description of what coping skills are, including a literature review illustrating the importance of coping skills. Next the section contains a discussion on a general model of coping for children and practical exercises in coping. The section concludes with specifics in applying the model to life circumstances that are troubling for many children.

Section II, Building Muscles for Mental Health, is focused on methods for promoting emotional well-being in children as a means of building their resources to meet the demands placed upon them. This section provides an understanding, grounded in research, of the cognitive and action strategies that promote emotionally healthy ways of thinking, living, and relating. The section also provides practical suggestions for counselors and mental health educators who want to implement educational programs that promote these skills for children in school and community settings. These skills include the child's knowledge of self, respect for self and others, healthy habit strength, and a balance between work and play.

Each of these two major sections of the book are self-contained and complete enough to be read independently and/or in any order. The contributing authors have attempted to speak to you as one voice in emphasizing the need for instruction in coping skills and mental health muscle.

The authors believe that preventing disorder and promoting health is a number one priority in our society today. An additional belief is that readers play a vital role in making preventive intervention a reality in their community.

The hope is that you will find this book helpful as you work with children in elementary schools and other community settings. Feedback and suggestions are welcomed as you try these ideas with the children in your community.

ACKNOWLEDGMENTS

Special appreciation is extended to many individuals and organizations who contributed to the preparation of *Empowering Children*.

The assistance of the contributing authors was vital to the completion of this book. Each of the contributing authors is a staff member of the Emotional Health Center, a prevention program within the Department of Psychiatry and Behavioral Sciences at the University of Oklahoma Health Sciences Center. Pamela Fischer, Ph.D., and Teresa Collins, M.A., researched and synthesized issues pertaining to special needs children. Marcy Price, M.A., edited several of the chapters. She also made several valuable suggestions in implementing various exercises in a more effective fashion.

Special thanks is also due to three public institutional systems who have supported this work. The Oklahoma State Department of Mental Health and Substance Abuse Services has supplied supporting funds to make prevention programming activities of the Emotional Health Center possible. The encouragement of the Department and, in particular, the support of Jan Hardwick, M.S.W., Director of Prevention Services, has been invaluable. Furthermore, the Oklahoma City Public Schools, Western Oaks Public Schools, and Putnam City Public Schools have welcomed and supported piloting of these exercises in their classrooms. Also, the Department of Psychiatry and Behavioral Sciences at the OU Health Sciences Center has housed the Emotional Health Center and provided staff and trainee support for prevention programming.

We would like to extend a special note of appreciation to the Feelings Factory and Virginia Boyter for allowing us to adapt and include material and artwork from the Enhancing Emotional Competence Curriculum.

Finally, we owe a special debt and thank you to Tania Jones, our Administrative Assistant, for her diligent typing, editing, and artistic contributions to this manuscript.

SECTION I
COPING SKILLS

Chapter 1

COPING

Mental health professionals and educators often believe that a part of their role in helping children is teaching them strategies for coping. They assert that children need to learn to cope with their emotions, adverse life situations, and various demands placed upon them. Yet, the word coping is used so frequently and in such a variety of contexts that it might be helpful to examine the meaning of coping more closely to achieve a common understanding.

In Webster's 21st Century Dictionary (1993, p. 66), coping is defined as "attacking or overcoming a problem or emergency." Synonyms for coping include "striving, dealing with, managing, handling, and facing" (Morehead, 1985, p. 106).

Lewis, Dlugokinski, Caputo, and Griffin (1988) believed that coping occurs when a person's resources for meeting demands exceed the demands placed upon them. When speaking of the ability to cope with one's personal emotional state, Irving Janis (1971) spoke of coping as the process of putting steps between what one feels and the resulting expression or action step taken. In this sense, then, coping is a process of incorporating a personal reaction to a difficult situation and subsequently expressing the feeling with constructive action.

Most individuals, then, view coping as successfully managing or handling difficulties. This fits with Caplan (1980) who spoke of coping as being related to the concept of competence. Caplan stated that

> Most researchers define competence as a system of learned attitudes and aptitudes, manifested as capacities for confronting, actively struggling with, and mastering life problems through the use of cognitive and social skills, and involving a capacity for resilience and perseverance in the face of emotional frustration and cognitive confusion. (p. 671)

An idea closely related to competency or the capacity to cope effectively is the concept of invulnerability. Rutter (1979) studied protective factors in children's responses to stress and environmentally disadvantaged situations. He discovered that, despite extremely adverse living conditions and social disadvantage, children can be well adjusted and even can develop an outstanding ability. These children, he said, were invulnerable to the stressors that might have caused other children to succumb to dysfunction or emotional disorder. Rutter's conclusions included the notion that invulnerability is a function of

> . . . compensating experiences outside the home, the development of self esteem, the scope and range of available opportunities, an appropriate degree of environmental structure and control, the availability of personal bonds and intimate relationships, and the acquisition of coping skills. (p. 70)

Therefore, children, who are viewed as competent or invulnerable, apparently have external or internal resources that mediate between the adverse conditions in their lives and their abilities or skills to moderate the impact of these conditions. By having the skills to cope effectively, these children are able to reduce their risk for developing disorders.

In an inclusive definition of coping skills, Hancock, Gager, and Elias (1993) incorporated the following attributes:

Self-Control Skills, which include the ability to listen carefully and accurately, follow directions, calm oneself down when under stress, and talk to others in a socially appropriate manner;

Social Awareness and Group Participation Skills, which focus on how to recognize and elicit trust, help, and praise from others, how to recognize others' perspectives, how to choose friends wisely, how to share, wait, and participate in groups, how to give and receive help and criticism, and how to understand others' perspectives; and

Social Decision Making and Problem Solving Skills, which involve an eight-step strategy to guide one in thoughtful decision making when facing health related and other personal and interpersonal choices or problematic situations, particularly when one is under stress.

The focus in this book is on coping as it relates to young children ages 5 through 11. Although Rutter's notion of invulnerability included both internal and external resources (1979), in this book, coping will be viewed as an internal resource that children can be taught in order to deal competently with the world. This internal resource includes the ability to recognize and deal with feelings and to develop constructive action tendencies in difficult life situations. This working definition of coping emphasizes the ability to persevere with constructive action toward healthy adjustment when emotionally aroused.

Coping, then, is a process. In this process the individual does not necessarily experience complete satisfaction or objective success. For example, coping effectively with emotional upheavals as a result of death or divorce means that individuals guide their own behavior in a series of constructive steps to adjust to difficulties that they face. It does not mean that their coping efforts objectively or subjectively negate the loss that they experience. Coping with an event, such as death or divorce, does not mean that the event or its impact is erased. Coping is the process of adjusting to that event in a healthy way.

Because coping with personal emotional arousal has been defined as the foundation of coping skills in young children, it may be helpful to look briefly at the nature of human emotions and their significance to our personal survival.

EMOTIONAL AROUSAL AND ITS SIGNIFICANCE IN COPING

Emotions ebb and flow in our lives because some events do matter to us. As long as we remain alive and responsive to the world in which we live, some of our experiences will carry a personal impact. When they do, we become emotional. Everyone of us has a uniqueness to our emotional life that is all our own. In this respect our emotions are unlike those of any other person; yet, at the same time, we experience similarities in our emotions. Some of those similarities (Dlugokinski, 1987) are described below.

Emotions Are Personal Adjustments to Change

When we become emotional, something about us is stirred up or changed. The word emotion originates from the Latin words *emovere* and *movere* and suggests a movement in our personal experience and approach. When we are frightened, our senses alert us to dangers and the need for flight. As we become angry, we mobilize reserve energy to fight or defend ourselves. In happiness or sadness we experience personal gains or losses and adjust our attitude accordingly. In an emotional state we are moved out of neutral.

Emotions Are Arousals of Mind and Body

Our mind and body work together in emotional arousal. Our body adapts through a series of changes in heart rate, muscle tension, breathing, and other physical adjustments. Our mind also adjusts by modifying thoughts and feelings to meet the changes as we perceive them. For example, when we are frightened, our body typically is in a state of vigilant response while we feel and think frightening thoughts. Furthermore, as we become angry, our mind and body work together to prime us to act in an assertive manner. If our anger is satisfactorily released, both our physical arousal and our angry thoughts and feelings will subside. If we only partially release it or express it in a way that magnifies the anger, then our tension continues.

Emotions Typically Are Aroused Involuntarily

In many circumstances, we become emotional instinctively. Our body changes and our thoughts and feelings shift involuntarily. The substance of these emotional adjustments is influenced by our association of past memories with current conditions. If we are mistreated by a bearded man with a cap, we may develop an intense fear reaction to beards or men who wear caps. Our initial emotional response to many situations is involuntary. In many instances, we do not have a choice of becoming emotional—our choice begins with what we do with those emotions.

While most authorities agree that emotions are involuntarily aroused, a multitude of popular misconceptions make recognition of our own emotional arousal difficult. Perhaps we learned that anger was a sign of disrespect, that fear was a sign of weakness, or that sadness was a sign of self-pity. Sexual and cultural stereotypes also can create problems. Thus, although our emotional arousal indeed may be involuntary, we may block out recognition for a variety of reasons. In doing so, we also are blocking our capacity to cope effectively.

Emotions Prepare Us to Act

When we are aroused emotionally, tension develops to release the arousal. When we are angry, we have urges within us to act in an angry manner. When we are happy, we also are aroused to express our happiness. Intense emotions commonly elicit some type of action. If we are sad, we may cry. If we are happy, we may smile or express our joy to others. If we are angry at others, we may act aggressively towards them or displace our anger, for example, by kicking a dog.

Although emotional arousal prepares us to act, it does not always result in action that is thoughtfully directed. Our tension may be released in a random activity or hyperactivity. Habits also may become automatic or thoughtless. For example, when we are angry we may habitually shout or throw objects. We do not think about being angry and expressing the anger; we just shout when we get angry. When we act without thought or awareness, we act impulsively.

Emotional tension also can be suppressed without behavioral expression. In such cases the tension may be absorbed in our body and result in physical distress. Headaches, stomachaches, and general physical tension often are associated with inadequate emotional release. Similarly, some of us may have a weak organ that constantly breaks down while others of us dispense our tensions more diffusely in our system. If we absorb a substantial amount of tension in our bodies, we can become prone to listlessness, apathy, or even clinical depression. Our body cannot stay in a stressful state forever without wearing down or losing steam.

Emotions Inform Us About Our Personal Condition

Our emotions mirror our experience of personal change; however, often we become emotional automatically and begin changing without realizing it. If we can become aware of the changes in our emotional condition, we can use the information for our personal benefit.

In pleasant emotions, the information is about an experience we enjoy. The feedback from our pleasant feelings is available for our memory and our learning. Through an awareness of the experience and the circumstances that helped it occur, we are more likely to repeat the incident, particularly if it does not bring added stress or accompanying unpleasant feelings.

Some immediately pleasant experiences, such as use of drugs or alcohol, are deceptively troublesome. They artificially alter our physiology and can hold long-term losses as consequences for momentary pleasantness. Many of our opportunities for experiencing beauty or joy, however, are not problematic. They are naturally pleasant if we take the time to notice them.

Pleasant experiences energize us. Noticing the beauty of a piece of art or a bird in flight enriches us. Recreation and relaxation give us reasons to endure more difficult moments. When we are informed about our joyful experiences, we can use these experiences to refresh ourselves.

Unpleasant emotions also provide information. They get our attention and mobilize us to consider alternate ways of living as we realize that our current approach is bringing us discomfort. The pain from touching a hot stove or casually handling a sharp knife can motivate us to become careful in our handling of objects that can hurt us. A fear of being struck by an automobile can help us become cautious as we enter a busy intersection. A sense of fear may mobilize us to run faster in an emergency. A sense of frustration may help us acquire new strength to overcome obstacles that are blocking us. Even a sense of sadness may help us deal with the reality of loss of a special person in our lives.

With an awareness of changes in our emotional condition, we can understand what is happening to us. We can acquire information about our personal condition and then use it to direct our own behavior. Our informed awareness can neither remove all pain from our lives nor make all things pleasant for us; however, awareness can help us reduce emotional tension or stress and, therefore, reduce unnecessary pain. It can help us savor our pleasant experiences and endure temporary discomfort.

ACQUIRING COMPETENCE IN COPING

Awareness of our emotions and of our choices for expression is a key to competence in coping. We acquire this awareness slowly as we become aware of ourselves and of our need to function independently. To trace that developmental acquisition we need to see the evolution of our emotionality from early stages of the life cycle to what is expected from us as competent adults.

Children do not learn this coping skill automatically. It is not something with which any of us are born. Rather, learning to cope with our feelings, frustrations, and difficulties is a developmental process, much like learning to walk, talk, or read. First, as infants, when we experience difficult emotions, our parents or other adults take responsibility for managing them for us. As very young infants, when we cry, we are usually fed, changed, or held by adults who try to soothe us. A little later, we may be allowed to cry for a few minutes. For example, if our parents are trying to establish our schedule of sleeping through the night they may endure five minutes of crying to test our ability to fall back to sleep. Even at this stage of development, we are being taught to forego the instant gratification of being fed or rocked or changed and instead learn to cope with our frustration and go back to sleep. The process of individuation has begun.

As we grow and mature, we take more and more responsibility for coping with our own emotions and life situations as the adults around us begin to relinquish their responsibility for managing them for us. It is hoped that, as adults, we will have learned our lessons in coping and will be able to function as responsible, mature persons who can impart our knowledge and experience about how to cope in our world to our own children.

The shift in responsibility is not an easy one. Sometimes we encounter difficult moments when others will not or cannot make us happy. As a result, we learn to cope in the best way we can. At times, parental urges to protect us as children linger long after we need them. At other times, as children, we also yearn for the earlier moments when our parents would fix everything for us. Sometimes the roles are reversed. As children we may feel responsible for the emotional welfare of our parents. When the responsibility for coping becomes blurred or fuzzy between two or more individuals, coping is adversely affected for all parties.

All of us have gaps in our own emotional development and lapses in our abilities to cope. We still may yearn to have somebody fix things for us when our emotions are unpleasant. We still may find some emotions difficult to accept. Sometimes we also seem to be bombarded by stressful changes that overwhelm us momentarily; however, we need to find ways to cope with our emotions in the best ways we can. Unless we remain protected all of our lives, our coping skills will determine whether our arousal will work for our personal welfare or in spite of it. We can learn to cope with our emotions most successfully by approaching them openly and with a sense of responsibility for our own emotional welfare.

COPING SKILLS INSTRUCTIONAL PROGRAMS

Much of the responsibility for teaching children to cope effectively is borne by parents and other significant adults. Within recent years, however, many instructional programs have been developed to teach children coping skills in elementary school settings. These programs are based on a multitude of methods, techniques, and theoretical orientations.

Compas, Banez, Malcarne, and Worsham (1991) reviewed the literature in an attempt to categorize the programs into fewer groups. Compas et al. (1991) concluded that these coping skills programs could be grouped into two main types, based on coping style emphasized in each program. One group of programs emphasizes problem-focused coping, which helps children learn effective ways of mastering aspects of persons, environment, or relationships between persons and environment that are perceived to be stressful. A second group of programs emphasizes emotion-focused coping, which typically teaches children to "manage or regulate the negative emotions associated with stressful episodes" (Compas et al., 1991, p. 27).

Problem-focused programs help children learn to think through their problems and to generate options and alternatives to solve difficult life situations. A good example of a coping skills program emphasizing problem-focused coping skills is the Interpersonal Cognitive Problem Solving (ICPS) Program (Shure & Spivack, 1982). This program was one of the first to be developed and serves as a model for many more recently developed programs (Denham & Almeida, 1987).

Unfortunately, very few instructional programs based on emotion-focused skills have been developed (Russner, Allen, Collins, & Dlugokinski, 1994). Those programs that educate children in emotion-focused coping generally emphasize building empathy and becoming sensitive to the emotional states of others.

A good example of an emotion-focused coping skills training program is Michelson's (1987) Behavioral Social Skills Training. This program develops interpersonal skills in the children including empathy, understanding others' rights, paying attention to others, and role taking. Other programs that incorporate feelings in their training include Weissberg, Caplan, and Sivo's (1989) Social Competence Program. In this program, however, understanding personal emotions are given only minor consideration in problem solving approaches.

Although the ICPS program and most emotion-focused programs devote some attention to teaching emotion-focused skills, the emphasis is placed on recognizing emotional states of *others* rather than on one's own emotional state. Yet, in a survey of the research on emotional sensitivity to others, Savitsky and Eby (1979) suggested that a limited connection exists between sensitivity to the emotions of others and the ability not to engage in antisocial, delinquent, or otherwise destructive behavior. They suggested that the individual perpetrator's inability to cope with persistent personal stress, emotional distress, and environmental demands is more likely to result in dysfunctional or disordered behavior.

The focus on others' emotional states is used by the ICPS program and many emotion-focused programs to aid in the decision-making process while trying to solve interpersonal problems. In these programs, however, an important self-management skill is neglected (Lazarus & Folkman, 1984). This skill, the ability to recognize and accept one's personal emotional state, is critical in the evolution of assuming personal responsibility for one's adjustment.

Other researchers also have demonstrated a strong connection between one's personal emotional state and overt behavior. Kashani, Deuser, and Reid (1991) found that high levels of unresolved anxiety may contribute to increased levels of verbal and physical aggression. In addition, Roberts (1988) reported that physically aggressive boys seem to have a blind spot for recognizing their own aggression. They are not in touch with their own emotional state.

Research suggests that the ability to solve problems and the ability to self-manage emotions tend to emerge at different stages of a child's development (Altshuler & Ruble, 1989; Band & Weisz, 1988; Wertlieb, Weigel, & Feldstein, 1987). Problem-focused skills seem to develop during pre- and early school years while sophisticated aspects of the ability to recognize one's own emotional state appears to develop in later childhood and early adolescence. This could be a result of the difficulty involved when young children try to observe and model adults who are managing an internal emotional state. Young children may be capable of early primitive emotional recognition and understanding, (i.e. the difference between happy and sad), but the nuances of more sophisticated emotions are beyond their grasp.

Despite the difficulty in learning this skill, children's ability to differentiate their own emotional state from the state of others plays a critical role in the development of a sense of personal responsibility. In a step-by-step process, children learn to build skills and to manage their own adjustment as they gradually begin to direct their own behavior. Because of the critical nature of this understanding, it is important, then, to educate children early about self-management of emotional states.

Pransky (1991) stated that children, even at an early age (e.g., ages 5 and 6), are able to delay their emotional responses a little. Later (e.g., ages 6 through 8), they begin to understand some issues in the cause and effect of their emotional responses. By ages 8 through 12, children can understand more abstract concepts related to emotions and their consequences. In this educational process, we need to be aware of these developmental differences in order to effectively reach children of differing ages and stages of development.

Educators and researchers have stressed the need for a comprehensive, school-based, coping skills program (Cowen, Hightower, Pedro-Carroll, & Work, 1990; Weissberg & Elias, 1993). This kind of program could include a generic approach to coping with a variety of stressful life situations and could be introduced in stages of complexity across the elementary school years. Different emphases each year could be based upon the developmental needs of children at each grade level.

The model proposed in this book for teaching children coping skills includes elements that can be introduced at varying degrees of complexity to match the developmental stage of the child. The model incorporates skills in personal emotional recognition, problem-solving, relaxation, and constructive action as part of the coping process. In tandem, we believe that these skills build emotional competence. Thus, we have named the model the ***Emotional Competence Model.*** This model also will include recognition of one's own emotional condition as a starting point for directing personal action and emotional expression in an appropriate manner. It is our belief that this understanding, acceptance, and ability to deal with one's emotional state is the foundation for personal adjustment and coping.

Chapter 2

THE EMOTIONAL COMPETENCE MODEL: A FOUR-STEP PROCESS FOR COPING

The Emotional Competence Model provides a framework for teaching children to cope with their own emotions and difficult life situations. The process of coping is accomplished in four steps or stages, and emotional competence is seen as the successful application of these steps in daily living. The model incorporates aspects of a "turtle technique" (Dlugokinski & Suh, 1989) with aspects of the problem-solving strategies of Myrna Shure and George Spivak (1982). It further incorporates relaxation exercises and ideas for body composure based on Arlene Koeppen's work (1974).

Historically, the Emotional Competence Program grew out of volunteer efforts with children and teachers in elementary schools. Both children and their teachers requested help for the children to learn to deal with their feelings. Volunteers were graduate students and faculty members in mental health, and they piloted various aspects of the coping steps in the Oklahoma City schools. The model evolved slowly over a period of several years. When the model was formalized into a curriculum, it became the official fourth-grade life skills education program of this urban school system.

The original curriculum uses animal imagery and puppets in a 30-session program (Dlugokinski & Suh, 1989). Turtles were chosen as main characters in the central story of the curriculum because they concretely illustrate steps of the model and are culturally sensitive. Pilot research on teaching children this four-step process has been promising. Instruction in a once-per-week, 45-minute format has been found to decrease children's aggressive choices in solving problems with a corresponding increase in nonviolent means of addressing difficult situations (Dlugokinski, Allen, Russner, Collins, & Fischer, 1994). Longitudinal research is needed to assess further the impact of this program and how it can be enriched with other classroom management, child empowerment, and family enrichment techniques. (Russner et al., 1994).

The Emotional Competence Model has been modified for reader convenience and use in this publication. The model's four-step process has been adapted to include two versions that are sensitive to both younger and older children. These adaptations were developed with sensitivity to developmental differences in emotion-focused coping skills and with consideration for the more primitive capacity of early elementary school children in this area. (Dubow, Schmidt, McBride, Edwards, & Merk, 1993). Furthermore, it has been modified to utilize human figures and characters instead of turtles as main characters in the various lessons. Although animal puppetry captures children's attention, puppets of this nature are not always accessible to counselors and mental health educators.

Although this four-step process is discussed here as a coping model for children, the same four steps are equally vital and helpful for adults (Dlugokinski, 1987). In fact, if adult teachers or counselors themselves do not understand or model this process, the material is likely to fail to have impact and to carry little meaning for children. To facilitate this modeling, considerable detail in examining the rationale for each coping step is included. The purpose is to have the reader to comprehend and demonstrate the coping technique with children in their daily lives.

In chapter 3 are included two separate, developmentally appropriate sets of sequential exercise programs to provide practice for children in the four coping steps. As a best choice, children would receive the first set of 20 exercises by the first or second grade (ages 5 through 7) and the second series a couple of years later (ages 8 through 11).

INTRODUCTION

Early in childhood, children begin developing their skills for thinking and acting independently. An integral part of this skill-building process is related to dealing with and gaining skills in managing difficult emotions. We help children develop their abilities as independent persons when we seize opportunities to help them progress towards managing their own emotions in a competent fashion.

As we assist children in learning skills to manage their own emotions, it is critical that we respect their individuality. Each of us has different kinds of issues that upset us or arouse us. When we become upset, we employ different styles for coping with difficulty. Some of us cope through withdrawal, some through physical activity, some through verbal expression or music. Because we enjoy different things, we experience pleasantness in different ways. Individual styles vary widely even within the same family. We need to respect children's individuality and help them find ways to cope that are suitable and helpful to them.

The Emotional Competence Model offers a way for coping that can be adapted to the individual style and issues of each person. Through a four-step process, the child arrives at a best choice. The best choice is the one "for me for now." It is not necessarily the person's best choice later or everyone's best choice. The best choice only has one basic guideline: It should not intentionally seek to harm the self or others.

In summary, the Emotional Competence Model for coping is based on four steps. Recognizing emotions is the first step. By ***accepting*** (Step I) our emotional arousals, we acquire an informed awareness about our personal condition. With this awareness, we then can ***pause*** (Step II) to collect ourselves and gain composure through relaxation. Then we can ***think*** (Step III) about our choices for emotional expression. In thinking, the third step, we get the big picture and consider our options in a thoughtful perspective. In the last step, we choose the best action available, and we ***do*** (Step IV) something to express our emotional tension. Each of these steps will be discussed in detail below.

UNDERSTANDING THE STEPS IN COPING

Step I. Accepting and Owning Our Emotional Arousals (Accept)

Many emotional experiences begin involuntarily as responses to personal change. By recognizing our emotions, we acquire the awareness we need to begin coping with them successfully.

Awareness of our emotional condition is far from automatic. Many of us have assigned deep-rooted meanings to our arousals that make ***acceptance*** and recognition difficult. Perhaps we learned that anger was a sign of disrespect or that fear was a sign of weakness. Maybe we grew up with a tradition of denying sadness or seeing it as self-pity. A variety of learned misconceptions can make it difficult for us to recognize and accept our emotional states.

Popular associations between emotionality and incompetence are all too common in our daily media exposure, and they exert a subtle but powerful pressure on us to deny our emotional condition. This kind of denial can lead us to a destructive spiral. By being unwilling to recognize our emotions or by being unable to accept them, we are prone to divert our tension into thoughtless activity, impulsive action, or bodily distress. Sometimes we attack others because we see them as the cause for bad or unacceptable feelings. By pretending that we are not aroused, we add new pressures and tensions to those already there.

If we block our emotions for long periods of time, we also can become apathetic, listless, or inert. We can turn off all emotionality as though nothing makes a difference to us. Our emotions are a source for vital energy. If we cut them off, we can become depressed and lose opportunities for pleasant emotions that help make life enjoyable.

To deny the existence of our emotional arousals is simply not dealing with reality; becoming emotional does not mean becoming dysfunctional. The healthy choice is to recognize and accept our emotions as a first step to coping with them. By recognizing them, we acquire an informed awareness about our personal condition.

The nature of this awareness becomes more sophisticated as we mature in our cognitive skills and personal experience. Our experience of simple discomfort branches out to more complex emotions of anger, fear, sorrow, jealousy, and guilt. As we acquire abstract thinking, we also experience more ambiguous anxieties and frustrations. On the pleasant side, our simple comforts diversify to security, love, joy, pride, and the appreciation of beauty. Each one of these emotions gives us feedback or information about our personal condition.

This feedback, however, is not always interpreted as information. As young children, our identity and sense of self is still primitive. We often believe that our unpleasant emotions result from a bad mother or father who do not give us what we want. Bad feelings come from others who do not take care of us. Good feelings come to us because others love us. Gradually, we can develop a sense of our own boundaries, improve our recognition and acceptance of our emotional condition, and attribute our emotional state to ourselves rather than to others. This learning is not quick or simple and often continues as a life-long process. Some individuals never acquire this skill.

We acquire the skills of emotional recognition and acceptance by becoming aware of ourselves as independent persons who have a responsibility for our personal condition. We learn to pay attention to changes in our own bodies as well as to changes in our thoughts and feelings. We recognize that this information is about our personal state. By learning to accept our emotions as a normal part of our lives, we can acquire what we need to cope with them in a successful way.

Step II. Pausing to Take Charge of Ourselves (Pause)

By recognizing our own emotional state, we set the stage for considering what to do with it in the context of our personal life. Particularly if we are uncomfortable, we feel a strong need to relieve the tension or discomfort. We recognize that we are angry, sad, frightened, or tense. Now what?

It would be simple to do whatever we feel like doing, or to do the first thing that comes to mind; however, it does not always make sense to release our emotions spontaneously. We could hurt ourselves or others. We sense that our impulses mean trouble. Our automatic ways of expressing ourselves will not help us. That is when we need to ***pause*** and to gain control of ourselves. Rather than an emotion controlling us, pausing allows us to choose to be in charge and to ask ourselves, "What am I going to do with me?"

Emotional tensions can be discharged temporarily by random actions or impulsive body movements. Random actions disrupt our concentration and attention. Impulsive actions may lead to violence. Without pausing to gain composure, we may act like pre-programmed robots automatically being taken somewhere we may not want to go. By releasing tension in this manner, we are likely to increase our problems.

As children learn to pause and to gain control of their bodies, they are more likely to act constructively on their own behalf. By sustaining a sense of body composure, children experience that they have a choice for body movement. As children gain body composure, they center, gather their energy, take charge, and provide direction for their own action. Pausing gives children an opportunity to gain the big picture by visualizing their choices from a realistic framework. They can begin to put their own energy to work for them.

Step III. Thinking About Our Options and Choices (Think)

The work in the first two steps sets the stage for problem-solving about how to direct our actions. Realistic choices can be discovered by considering our emotional condition within a larger perspective. By taking the time to ***think,*** we gain a perspective and see the big picture of what we can do to release our emotions in a constructive way. To get this big picture, we need information about our personal and environmental conditions in order to visualize our choices from a realistic framework.

The ability to consider choices for our own actions does not appear overnight. Its roots lie in our earliest experiences of thinking for ourselves and believing that the power of our own actions can make a difference. As we nurture these qualities, practice them, and refine them, we improve our abilities to consider appropriate actions in our lives. We begin to believe and to act as if we have the right to make intelligent decisions. When those decisions are wrong, we have a right to learn from our mistakes. Our ability to think about our choices helps us cope with difficulty, but it also affects our capacity to enjoy pleasant experiences. Thinking for ourselves is our self-management system, our opportunity to plan ways to enjoy and to take care of ourselves. By planning ways to experience pleasant times and to cope with unpleasant ones, we need not become overwhelmed by either of them.

The effectiveness of our thought process depends on the *kind of information* that we consider and the *way* in which we consider it. Realistic information is our data base for exploring effective options. We need to feed our minds with the facts of our current situation in order to put the facts into a meaningful perspective. With that perspective, we then can play with our possible choices.

The manner in which we consider information about our situation is also critical. If we are centered, we can concentrate on directing our own actions rather than on trying to manipulate others. This gives us the greatest opportunity for effective deliberation.

Several strategies that can help us in centering, thinking through, and selecting appropriate options are listed below:

Thinking in the first person: I am considering my options for action. I need my brain to focus on what is possible for me. "I" is a self-organizing pronoun that helps me think without becoming fragmented. By thinking in the first person, "I" can plan my approach, what "I" will do. "I" can commit my energy to a choice I make.

Reviewing current circumstances: My initial emotional arousal is often involuntary and may be connected to old memories and habits. My current situation may fit those old memories, or it may not. What is my setting and situation? Choices perfectly suitable for me in some situations are inappropriate for me in others. Am I in a church, my home, a playground, or in the classroom? My response may need to vary in each circumstance.

Establishing priorities: Where am I going and what is the most important thing for me to consider? What can wait? What cannot wait? When I am emotional, I can become confused and scattered. Important issues can get lost and overwhelmed by items that grab my immediate attention. I can get a realistic perspective of my current priorities by "collecting myself" and giving the critical issues my priority attention.

Reviewing personal limitations and capabilities: In my present emotional state what can I do? What am I unable to do? Where do I need support? What is an honest yet realistic response for me at the present time?

Looking ahead to the consequences of options: No one can fully predict the future, but I can make educated guesses by visualizing what is likely to happen. My personal actions are connected to other events in my future. If I do this, then that is likely to happen. If I do that, then this is more likely. *If-then thinking* is a way for me to sort through my possible actions and imagine likely results. I become playful with what my future might look like.

Valuing myself and others: When I am respecting myself and others simultaneously, my choice is most likely to work. It is based on a principle of fairness and compassion. Sometimes there is a tendency to consider only myself or only others. Both deserve a caring consideration.

Step IV. Acting on Our Best Choice (Do)

By expressing an emotional state, we release the tension that has aroused us. Deliberate expression means acting upon the best choice for us at the present time. This choice is most effective when it is respectful of ourselves and others simultaneously. By thoughtfully choosing to do something, we do the best we can do for now. We and others need to be respected. Our best choice may not always be ideal, but it is the best choice available for now.

Sometimes it is easy for us to get stuck in thinking about the very best or perfect thing to do. We all would like a guarantee that we are not making a mistake. Yet often there are no correct answers and no ways to avoid taking some kind of risk. Our best choice for now is the best we can do. If it is a mistake, we can learn from it and make a better choice next time. At least it is our own choice, one we have considered to the best of our ability.

Sometimes verbally expressing an emotion is a constructive way of coping with it. For example, saying "I am sad" or "I am afraid" can bring us empathy and social support. By telling someone "I am angry," we assert ourselves. We assert our feeling that someone may have been unfair to us. Our expression also brings the source of our discomfort to their awareness, but without blaming them for it. When we are able to own our thoughts and feelings and express them from a perspective of "I think" or "I feel," we retain our boundaries and maximize the opportunities that we have to be listened to. When both parties remain open to this kind of healthy expression and listening, problems are more likely to be resolved. Even if the problem is not resolved per se, some tension is released in the simple expression. In a conscious expression of anger, we express ourselves about a specific incident of personal aggravation and keep our personal boundaries. We do not get lost in a name-calling power struggle or attack others impulsively.

Sometimes, however, such as in the presence of abusive or alcoholic parents, expressing an emotion verbally may not be appropriate. Such an expression may lead to destructive or abusive consequences. The circumstances and likely consequences need to be considered in order to make our best choice a realistic one.

When social understanding is not required or support is not realistic, nonverbal expression may be sufficient. By looking ahead momentarily to the likely consequences of our actions, we might discharge the tension of our emotions with constructive actions. For example, a majority of us report that we feel better after we have a good cry. Crying may release the tensions and sadness we feel during times of loss. At other times, perhaps listening to music or going for a walk might help.

Physical activity also can help us break the grip of uncomfortable emotional states. A vibrant walk, a physically active game, or a fantasy boxing match with a punching bag can help us cope with anger or depression. Aerobic activity with deep breathing is particularly helpful. It seems to cleanse our system and help us put things into perspective. Coping effectively with anger may sometimes even mean fighting. In such cases, fighting is a conscious choice, not an impulsive reckless gesture.

We can improve the likelihood that our best choice will be implemented when we take action for today, one step at a time. For now, for this day, this action makes sense. Taking only one step at a time makes it possible for us to begin doing something rather than to remain riddled with conflict or indecision. Similarly, if our actions need to be modified, we can change them without having to make major readjustments. We think about what is best for now, and then act in small steps.

SUMMARY

In the Emotional Competence Model, coping is viewed as the business of recognizing emotional pain and managing emotional arousals. Practicing the four coping steps—accepting, pausing, thinking, and doing—habitually and consistently is empowering. Daily practice of this coping strategy provides the strength and skill to enhance emotional welfare and life satisfaction.

Chapter 3

PRACTICAL EXERCISES IN COPING

The framework proposed in this book for educating children in coping skills has four steps. Each step requires learning a separate skill that needs to be integrated into a total picture. The three introductory exercises in this chapter integrate these skills into a big picture to help the children remember the four coping steps. The methods used to incorporate these four separate skills into a larger whole include the use of a story, a song, and a words-to-rhythm jingle.

Stories present ideas in a nurturing way. Children look forward to having the same stories told to them over and over again. Sometimes the repetition itself helps children feel a sense of security and predictability. The story in Introductory Exercise 1, *Tom and Jeri Learn to Cope,* was developed to introduce and to integrate the four coping steps. The recommended procedure is to read the story to the children as an introduction to the coping process, followed by having them do a detailed review of the major ideas presented in the story in each of the three introductory exercises. Briefer reviews can be included in the remainder of the exercises.

Songs and jingles also can provide a fun way to learn and remember important themes. A song has a way of staying with us and becoming a part of our long-term memory. We can access its message for our enjoyment or in times of trouble. The message of both the song and the jingle help children see the big picture of how the four coping steps can help them. The song, *Accept My Feelings Inside,* is written into the story itself. The words-to-rhythm jingle, *Reason 'n Rhyme,* is included as a third introductory exercise to this coping skills education program. Recordings of the song and the words-to-rhythm jingle are included on the accompanying audiotape. Sheet music of the song and jingle are located in Figures 3.1., 3.2., and 3.3.

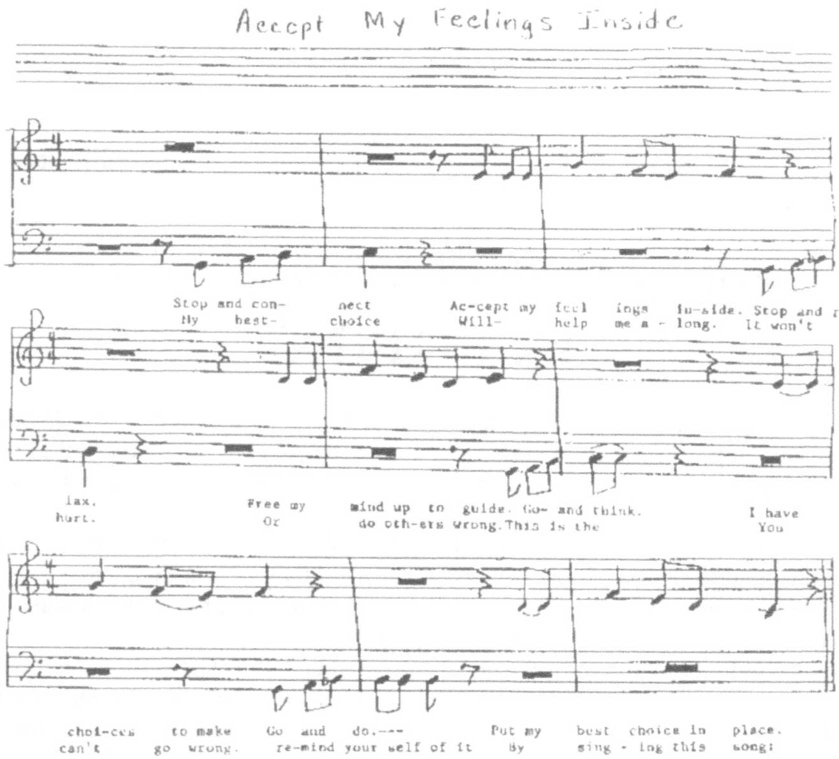
Accept My Feelings Inside
Stop and con- nect Ac-cept my feel ings in-side. Stop and re
My best- choice Will- help me a - long. It won't
lax. Free my mind up to guide. Go- and think. I have
hurt. Or do oth-ers wrong. This is the You
choi-ces to make Go and do.--- Put my best choice in place.
can't go wrong. re-mind your self of it By sing - ing this song:

Figure 3.1. Sheet music for *Accept My Feelings Inside*. Permission is granted to enlarge and photocopy for classroom use.

Reason 'n Rhyme
Chorus

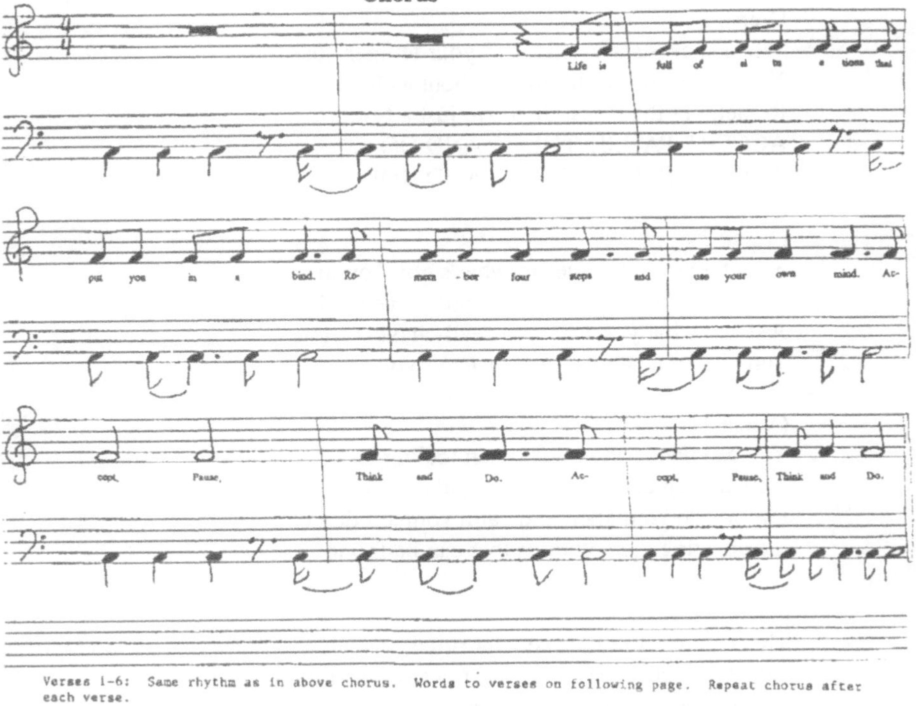
Life is full of si tu a tions that
put you in a bind. Re- mem - ber four steps and use your own mind. Ac-
cept, Pause, Think and Do. Ac- cept, Pause, Think and Do.
Verses 1-6: Same rhythm as in above chorus. Words to verses on following page. Repeat chorus after each verse.

Figure 3.2. Sheet music for *Reason 'n Rhyme* chorus. Permission is granted to enlarge and photocopy for classroom use.

Reason 'n Rhyme

(Verse 1)
When sparks start to fly, and your temper does too,
You're headin' for trouble without a clue,
Remember the steps, there are just a few,
ACCEPT, PAUSE, THINK, AND DO . . .
ACCEPT, PAUSE, THINK, AND DO!

(Verse 2)
Your feelings are clues to what's goin' on inside,
Learn to listen to them, you don't have to hide.
Just say what you feel, you really have a choice,
Tune in for a change to your inner voice.

(Verse 3)
You can pause and relax when feeling bad,
Take a deep breath if you're mad or sad.
Pull inside your shell and calm yourself down,
It's amazing the solutions that can be found.

(Verse 4)
Think, think, think—use your mind,
Come up with ideas that won't put you in a bind.
Good ideas, that won't hurt anyone,
Search for answers, then you're almost done.

(Verse 5)
It's time to take some action, make a move that's right for you,
Rely on heart and head, not the ol' one-two!
No one wins when the fists go flyin',
Depend on your brain, and you won't be cryin'.

(Verse 6)
Accept the way you feel, and then count to ten,
Put your mind to the test, and then begin,
Think about your options, and which of them is right,
Then take a stand, hold with all of your might.

(Chorus) (Repeat chorus after each verse)
Life is full of situations that put you in a bind,
Remember four steps, and use your own mind . . .
ACCEPT, PAUSE, THINK, AND DO . . .
ACCEPT, PAUSE, THINK, AND DO!

Figure 3.3. Lyrics to words-to-rhythm jingle, *Reason 'n Rhyme*. Permission is granted to enlarge and photocopy for classroom use.

INTRODUCTORY EXERCISES 1 THROUGH 3

Objective

To help children learn, integrate, and remember the four steps for coping with their emotions and difficult life situations.

The following three exercises have been developed for use as an introduction to the coping skills instruction program. They are designed both for 5- through 7-year-olds and 8- through 11-year-olds.

INTRODUCTORY EXERCISE 1. TOM AND JERI LEARN TO COPE

Activity

Read or tell in detail the following story to the children. After completing the story, ask the children to remember with you major segments of the story. The song in the story is put to music on an accompanying audiotape and on sheet music located at the end of this chapter. Play the song for the children after you have read the story to them.

"Tom and Jeri Learn to Cope"

Tom and Jeri are friends. Most of the time they enjoy playing together. Something happens every week, though, that spoils Tom and Jeri's playtime.

Tom likes to play soccer. It is his favorite game. He always wants to play soccer with Jeri. So, once or twice a week he asks Jeri to kick the ball with him in his backyard. Tom always likes to practice his kicking.

Jeri does not like soccer at all. She feels hurt that Tom asks her to play soccer over and over again when he knows that she does not like to play it.

Jeri always makes up a reason to go home when Tom suggests playing soccer. Then Tom gets angry and calls Jeri names. He says things like "Baby, baby, you are a baby. You can't kick the ball. That's why you don't want to play."

Tom sometimes feels sad that Jeri will not play soccer with him, and Jeri feels hurt and angry with Tom when he calls her names. When they get upset with each other, they miss the special fun they both enjoy in playing together.

One day Tom's Grandpa Jim heard Tom call Jeri a name. He saw Jeri running home. Grandpa Jim asked Tom and Jeri to come talk to him about what happened.

Tom explained that he loved soccer and that he felt really angry when Jeri would not play. Grandpa Jim said that he understood how Tom felt. Then Jeri explained to Grandpa Jim that she did not feel that a *real* friend would ask you to play a game that he *knew* you didn't like. Grandpa Jim said he understood.

Then Grandpa Jim said, "I learned something as a boy from my Grandmother Ruth that helped me then and helps me now. It helps me most when I feel angry, sad, or hurt about something. It could help you, Tom, and you, Jeri, when you feel angry or hurt. Grandmother Ruth taught me this little song to help me deal with my feelings. It's called *Accept My Feelings Inside*.

"Accept My Feelings Inside"

Stop and connect!
Accept my feelings inside.
Stop and relax!
Free my mind up to guide.

Go and think!
I have choices to make.
Go and do!
Put my best choice in place.

My best choice
Will help me along.
It won't hurt
Or do others wrong.

This is the secret.
You can't go wrong.
Remind yourself of it
By singing this song.

Then Grandpa Jim said, "Just remember: ACCEPT, RELAX, THINK, AND DO. That's the way to keep control of you."

After talking with Grandpa Jim, Tom and Jeri walked home and started singing the song to themselves. Sometimes they sang it together. They remembered the song from Grandpa Jim and the messages in the song. They talked about their feelings with each other. They thought of ways of playing that would be good for both of them. Sometimes they played soccer. Sometimes they played other games. They decided they could find ways to be together and have fun.

INTRODUCTORY EXERCISE 2. ACCEPT MY FEELINGS INSIDE

Activity

Review the major themes of the story, *Tom and Jeri Learn to Cope*. Consider having the children read the story themselves or role-play the story. Roles could include a narrator, Grandpa Jim, Tom, and Jeri.

Use the last half of the session to teach the children the song, *Accept My Feelings Inside*. Consider making copies of the sheet music (Figure 3.1) for the children to help them learn the song.

Play the song through once (located on the accompanying audiotape) and have the children simply listen to the words and music. Play it through again, stopping after each verse and have the children sing the verse with you. End the session by having the children sing through the entire song accompanied by the audiotape version.

INTRODUCTORY EXERCISE 3. REASON 'N RHYME

Activity

Sing the song, *Accept My Feelings Inside,* accompanied by the audiotape.

Briefly review the main themes of the story again, focusing on the emotions the characters were feeling.

Tell the children that Grandpa Jim decided to give Tom and Jeri another way to remember the four coping steps. Then play the words-to-rhythm jingle, *Reason 'n Rhyme,* located on the accompanying audiotape and in Figures 3.2 and 3.3.

Play it again, this time stopping at the end of each stanza to allow the children to say the words with you.

To help the children learn the words, consider making copies of the words to *Reason 'n Rhyme*.

INTEGRATING THE FOUR-STEP COPING PROCESS INTO THE REMAINING EXERCISES

An effective procedure is to review the story and sing the song at the beginning of each remaining exercise. As a way of closing each exercise, say the words-to-rhythm jingle. The story, song, and jingle integrate the four coping steps—accept, pause, think, and do—in an easy-to-remember format.

The children can be helped by a visual reminder of the Four Steps to Coping that they learn in the song and jingle. One way to incorporate this reminder is to have the children illustrate each verse of the words-to-rhythm jingle, *Reason 'n Rhyme*. Another fun exercise is to have the children make a poster, classroom book, or mural illustrating with their own artwork the four major themes in the song and jingle. Those themes could be as follows:

I Can . . .

Accept: Know My Feelings Inside.
Pause: Let My Mind Be My Guide.
Think: I Have Choices to Make.
Do: Put My Best Choice in Place.

PRACTICAL EXERCISES FOR STEP I—ACCEPT

Accept.
Stop and connect!
Recognize my feelings inside.

Objective

To help children develop awareness and acceptance of their own feeling states and situations where those feelings may occur.

Recognizing and accepting feelings is the first step toward gaining control of them. If children are not taught to know what they feel, they are likely to be headed toward action that will not help them—action that may be destructive to themselves or others. This action often leads to harmful consequences. Putting words to feelings and naming them is often the first step in understanding and accepting them.

The following pages include some practical exercises designed to help children recognize and accept their feelings. Five acceptance exercises have been written for 5- through 7-year-old children, and five have been written for 8- through 11-year-old children.

STEP I, EXERCISE 1. FEELINGS HAVE NAMES (Ages 5 Through 7)

Materials

- Magazines (if possible, one for each child)
- Tape, glue, or paste
- Scissors

Activity

Explain to the children that sometimes we can guess what people are feeling by looking at expressions on their faces. We also have different expressions on our faces when our feelings change. Explain that these feelings have names.

Have the children cut four pictures out of magazines. Tell them to choose two pictures where the people look happy and two pictures where they look unhappy. Ask the children to paste their pictures on a sheet of paper and write happy or unhappy under each picture. If the children are not able to write, have them draw symbols under their picture of happy (☺) or unhappy (☹).

Then have the children share with the class what their pictures may depict. Tell the children to make up or create a brief story about why they think this person is happy or unhappy.

If time permits, have the children talk about one time that they felt happy and unhappy.

STEP I, EXERCISE 2.
FEELINGS CAN BE HAPPY OR UNHAPPY
(Ages 5 Through 7)

Materials

- Two 8 1/2" x 11" sheets of white paper are needed—one with the word and visual image of HAPPY (☺) on it, the other with the word and visual image of UNHAPPY (☹) on it.
- Feelings pictures are located in Figures 3.4, 3.5, and 3.6. Photocopy and separate the pictures by cutting them on the dotted lines.

Activity

Put the two sheets of white paper on the floor or bulletin board where all the children can see them. Tell the children that some of the feelings we have are happy (i.e., feel good) whereas others are unhappy (i.e., feel bad).

Hold up the feelings pictures one at a time. Ask the children, as a group, to look at the feelings pictures, and to decide, as a group, whether the feeling depicted on the child's face is happy or unhappy. After the group decides, place or pin the picture by the paper that says *happy* or the one that says *unhappy.* Be sure that all the pictures can be seen simultaneously so that you have two collages of faces, *happy* and *unhappy.*

After all the pictures are placed, ask, "What could make someone happy?" "What could make someone unhappy?" Take several answers and allow time for discussion.

Sometimes children only focus on what others can do to make someone feel happy or unhappy. They neglect that they can do things to make themselves feel happy or unhappy. If time permits, ask the children to talk about and draw the things they can do to make themselves feel happy or unhappy.

Suggestion: Put the drawings on a bulletin board in the classroom with appropriate pictures surrounding the words "I am happy" and "I am unhappy" as a reminder to the children of the feelings and situations that were discussed.

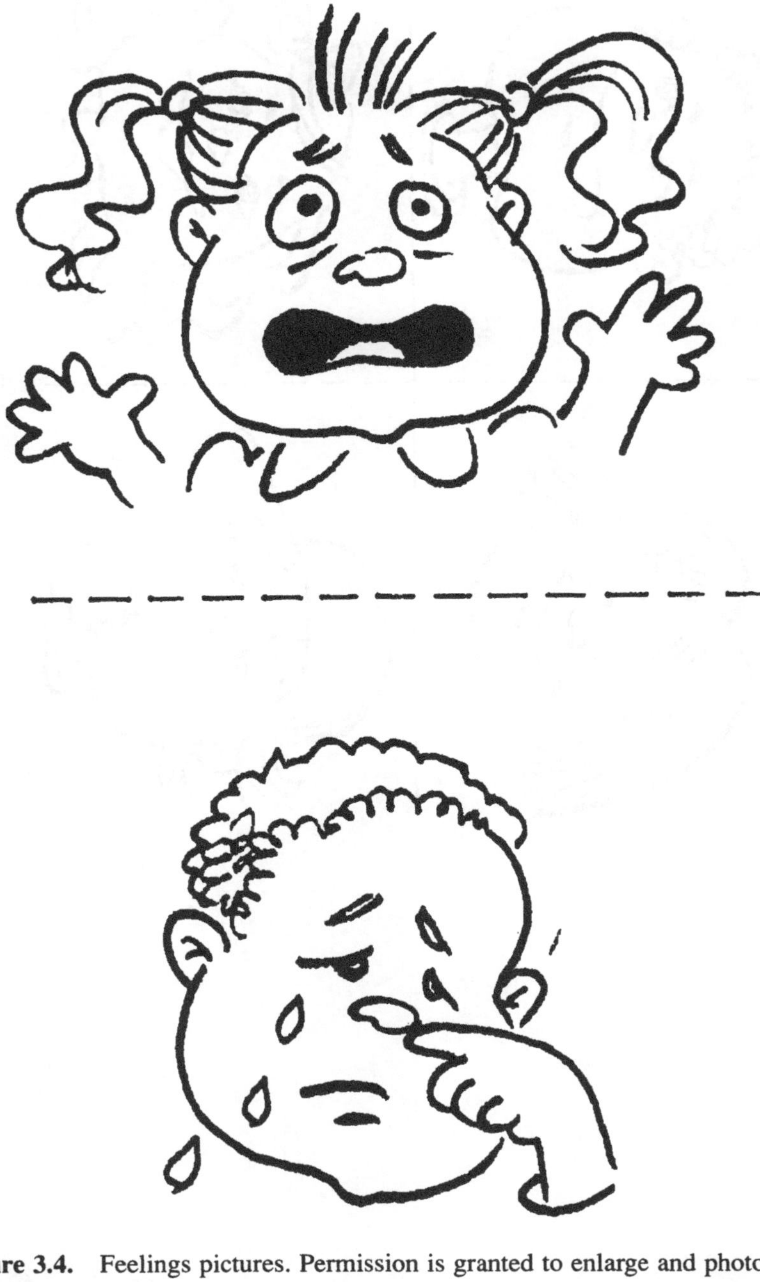

Figure 3.4. Feelings pictures. Permission is granted to enlarge and photocopy for classroom use.

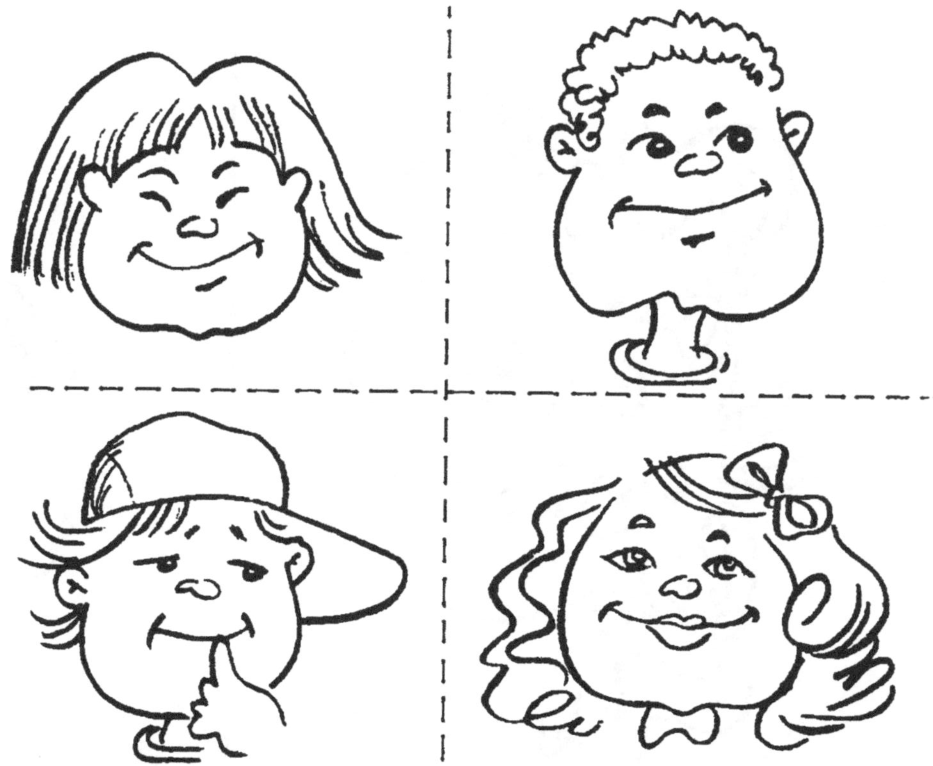

Figure 3.5. Feelings pictures, Continued. Permission is granted to enlarge and photocopy for classroom use.

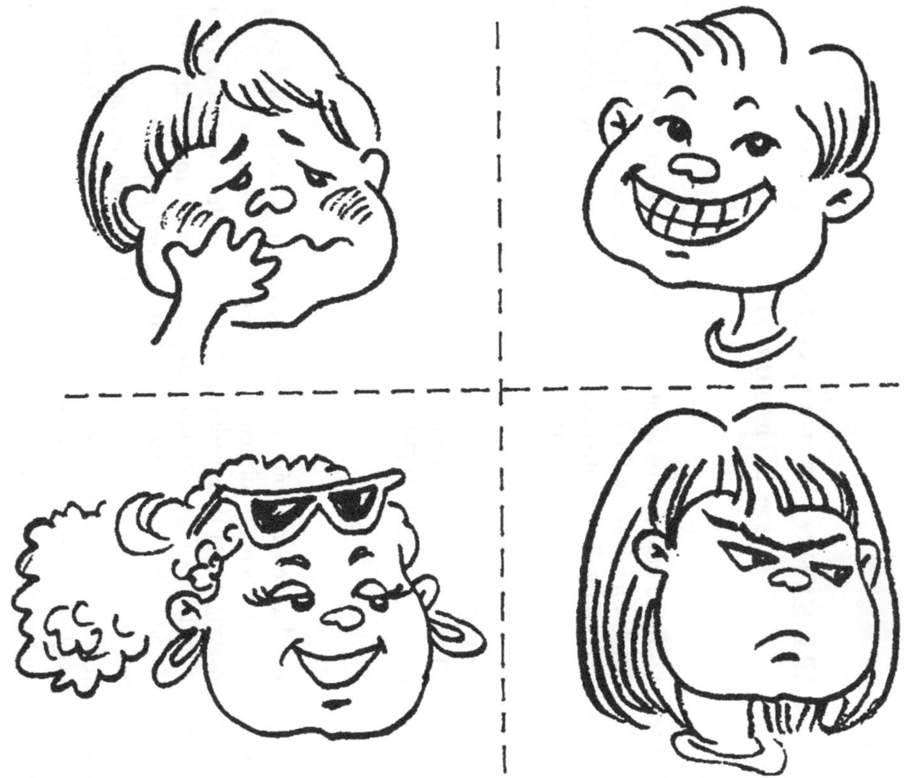

Figure 3.6. Feelings pictures, Continued. Permission is granted to enlarge and photocopy for classroom use.

STEP I, EXERCISE 3. I HAVE FEELINGS (Ages 5 Through 7)

Materials

- The feelings listed here can be located on cards in Figures 3.7, 3.8, 3.9, and 3.10. Photocopy and cut the cards apart so that each can be held up separately. (A culturally sensitive, colorful set of these feeling cards can be purchased through The Feelings Factory, Raleigh, NC, 1-800-858-2264.)

HAPPY	SAD
SATISFIED	ANGRY
PROUD	ASHAMED
SAFE	FRIGHTENED

- A rubber ball

Activity

Tell the children that you are going to hold up a card (e.g., happy) and say a word out loud that describes how children sometimes feel.

Read a brief description of that feeling as found on the feelings card. Then ask for a volunteer to describe what children might do or what might happen to children that could lead to their feeling that way. Take several examples.

Repeat the same procedure (i.e., reading and discussion) with the sad card.

If the children only talk about things others do that cause certain feelings, you occasionally might ask the question, "What can children themselves do that might cause them to feel happy? Sad?"

If the sophistication of the group permits, continue in the same way with the rest of the list.

If time permits, have the children sit in a big circle. Have one child hold a ball and say, "I feel happy when I _________ ," completing the sentence with a situation to accompany this feeling. Then ask the child to roll the ball to another child in the circle. Have the second child complete the same sentence with another situation. Repeat the above with other children or other feelings as time permits. (Try to include happy and sad at a minimum.)

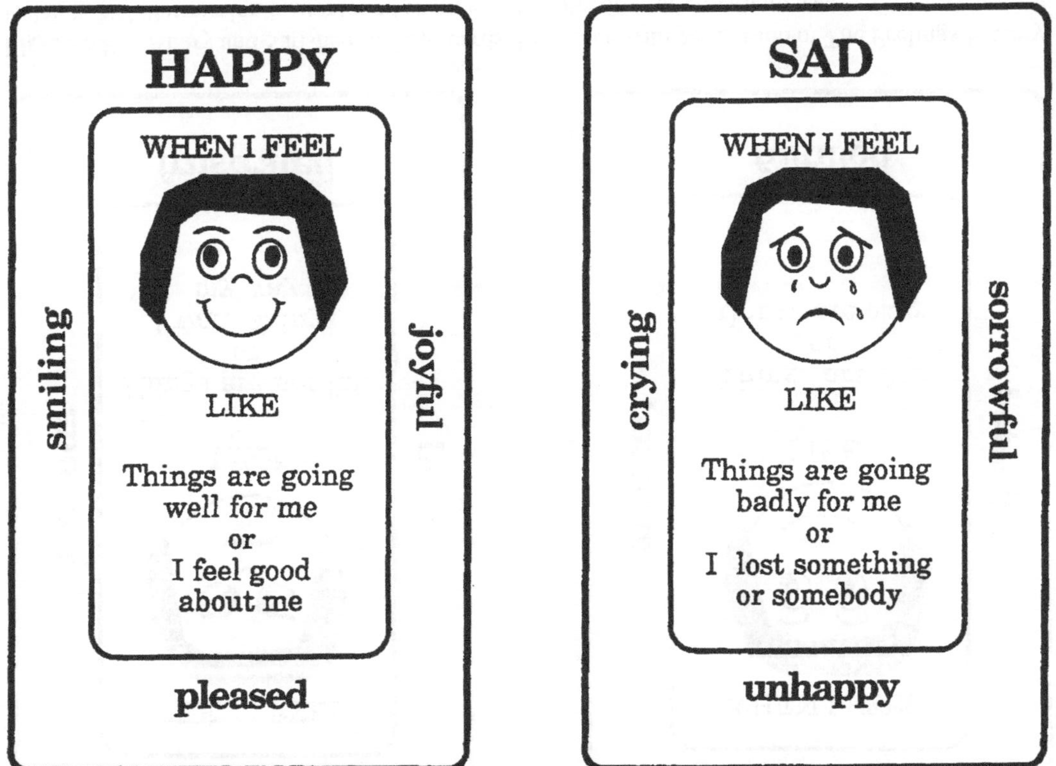
HAPPY
WHEN I FEEL
LIKE
Things are going well for me or I feel good about me
smiling
joyful
pleased
SAD
WHEN I FEEL
LIKE
Things are going badly for me or I lost something or somebody
crying
sorrowful
unhappy

Figure 3.7. Happy and Sad feelings cards. Reprinted with permission of The Feelings Factory, Raleigh, NC. Permission is granted to enlarge and photocopy for classroom use.

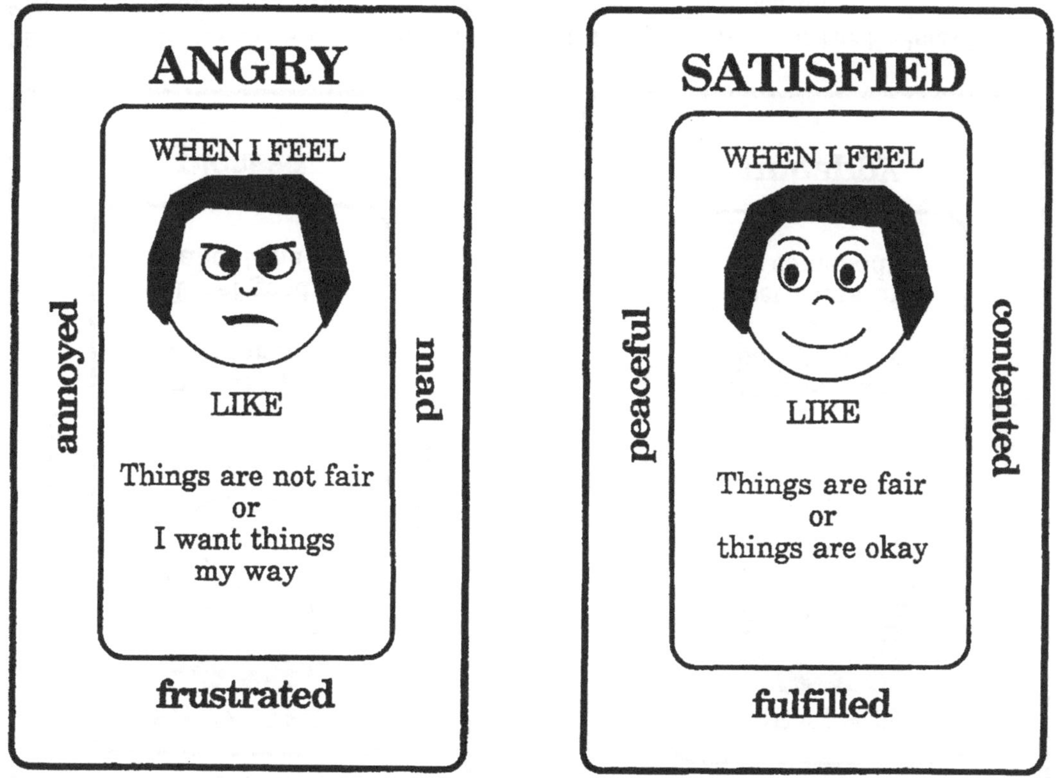
ANGRY
WHEN I FEEL
LIKE
Things are not fair
or
I want things
my way
annoyed
mad
frustrated
SATISFIED
WHEN I FEEL
LIKE
Things are fair
or
things are okay
peaceful
contented
fulfilled

Figure 3.8. Angry and Satisfied feelings cards. Reprinted with permission of The Feelings Factory, Raleigh, NC. Permission is granted to enlarge and photocopy for classroom use.

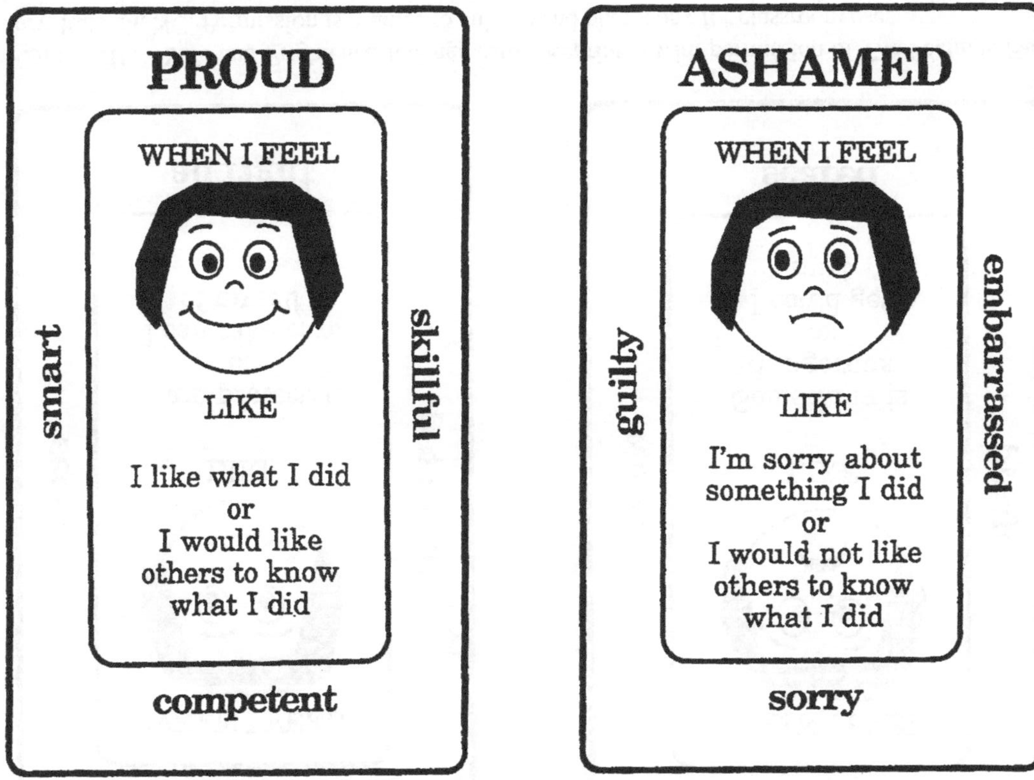
PROUD
WHEN I FEEL
LIKE
I like what I did
or
I would like
others to know
what I did
smart
skillful
competent
ASHAMED
WHEN I FEEL
LIKE
I'm sorry about
something I did
or
I would not like
others to know
what I did
guilty
embarrassed
sorry

Figure 3.9. Proud and Ashamed feelings cards. Reprinted with permission of The Feelings Factory, Raleigh, NC. Permission is granted to enlarge and photocopy for classroom use.

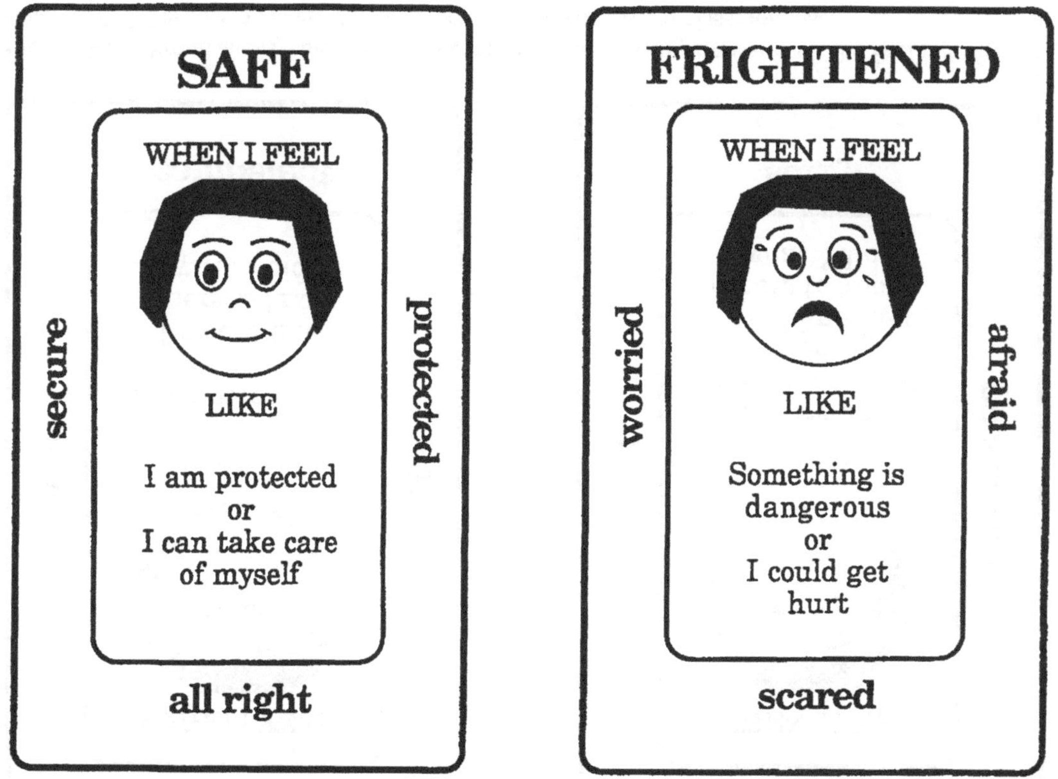
SAFE
WHEN I FEEL
LIKE
I am protected
or
I can take care
of myself
secure
protected
all right
FRIGHTENED
WHEN I FEEL
LIKE
Something is
dangerous
or
I could get
hurt
worried
afraid
scared

Figure 3.10. Safe and Frightened feelings cards. Reprinted with permission of The Feelings Factory, Raleigh, NC. Permission is granted to enlarge and photocopy for classroom use.

STEP I, EXERCISE 4. I HAVE FEELINGS, Continued (Ages 5 Through 7)

Materials

- The following feelings are located on cards in Figures 3.11, 3.12, 3.13, and 3.14. Photocopy and separate the cards on the dotted lines.

LOVE	HATE
INTERESTED	BORED
BELONGING	LONELY
RELAXED	NERVOUS

- A rubber ball

Activity

Tell the children that you are going to hold up a card (e.g., love) and say a word out loud that describes how children sometimes feel.

Read a brief description of that feeling as found on the feelings card. Then ask for a volunteer to describe what children might do or what might happen to children that could lead to their feeling that way. Take several examples.

Repeat the same procedure with the word hate.

If the children only talk about things others do that cause certain feelings, you occasionally might ask the question, "What can children themselves do that might cause them to feel love? Hate?

If the sophistication of the group permits, continue in the same way with the rest of the list.

If time permits, repeat the final activity—the rubber ball roll—described in Exercise 3.

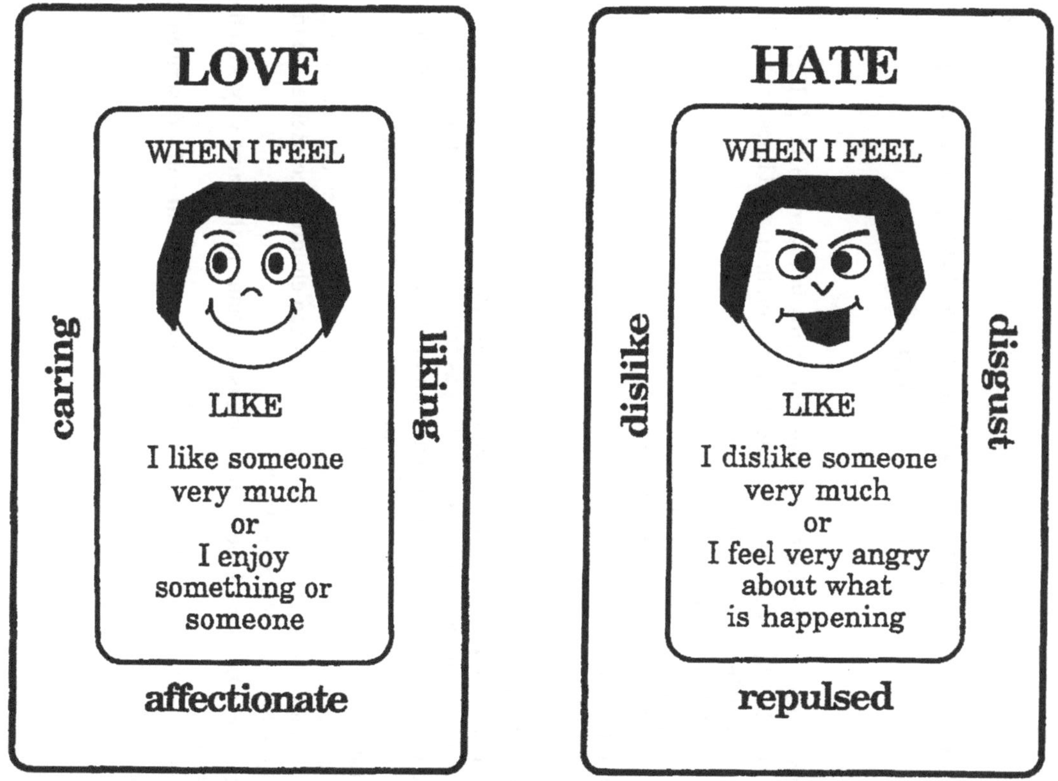
LOVE
WHEN I FEEL
LIKE
I like someone very much or I enjoy something or someone
caring
liking
affectionate
HATE
WHEN I FEEL
LIKE
I dislike someone very much or I feel very angry about what is happening
dislike
disgust
repulsed

Figure 3.11. Love and Hate feelings cards. Reprinted with permission of The Feelings Factory, Raleigh, NC. Permission is granted to enlarge and photocopy for classroom use.

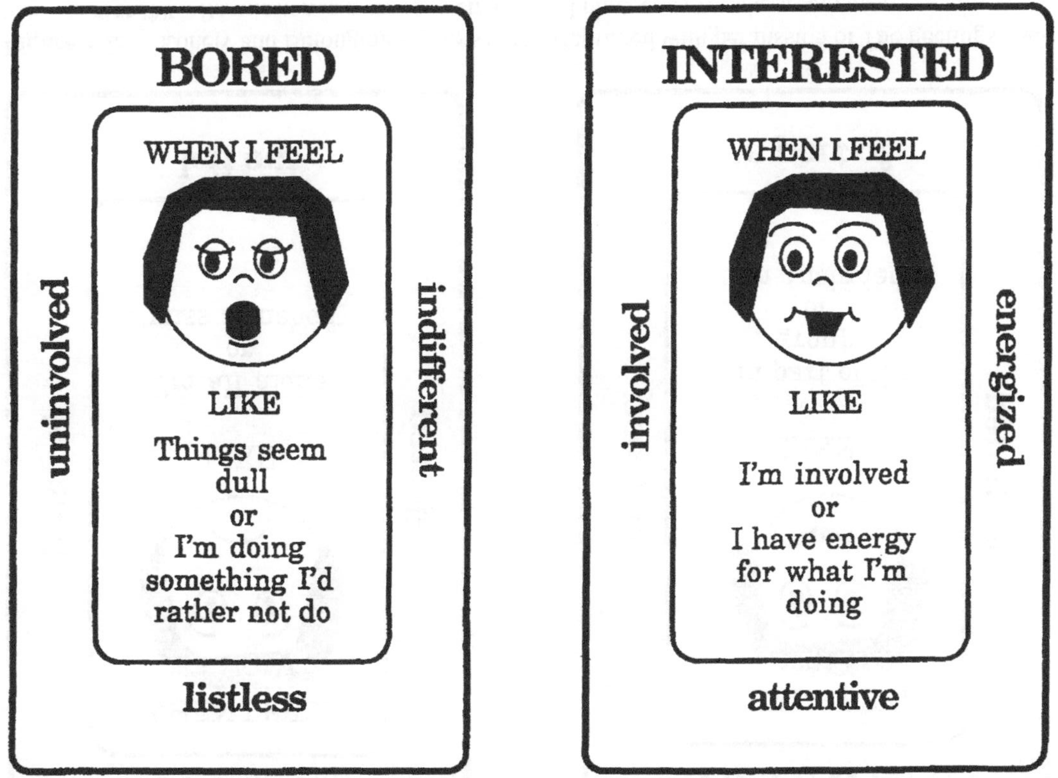
BORED
WHEN I FEEL
LIKE
Things seem dull or I'm doing something I'd rather not do
uninvolved
indifferent
listless
INTERESTED
WHEN I FEEL
LIKE
I'm involved or I have energy for what I'm doing
involved
energized
attentive

Figure 3.12. Bored and Interested feelings cards. Reprinted with permission of The Feelings Factory, Raleigh, NC. Permission is granted to enlarge and photocopy for classroom use.

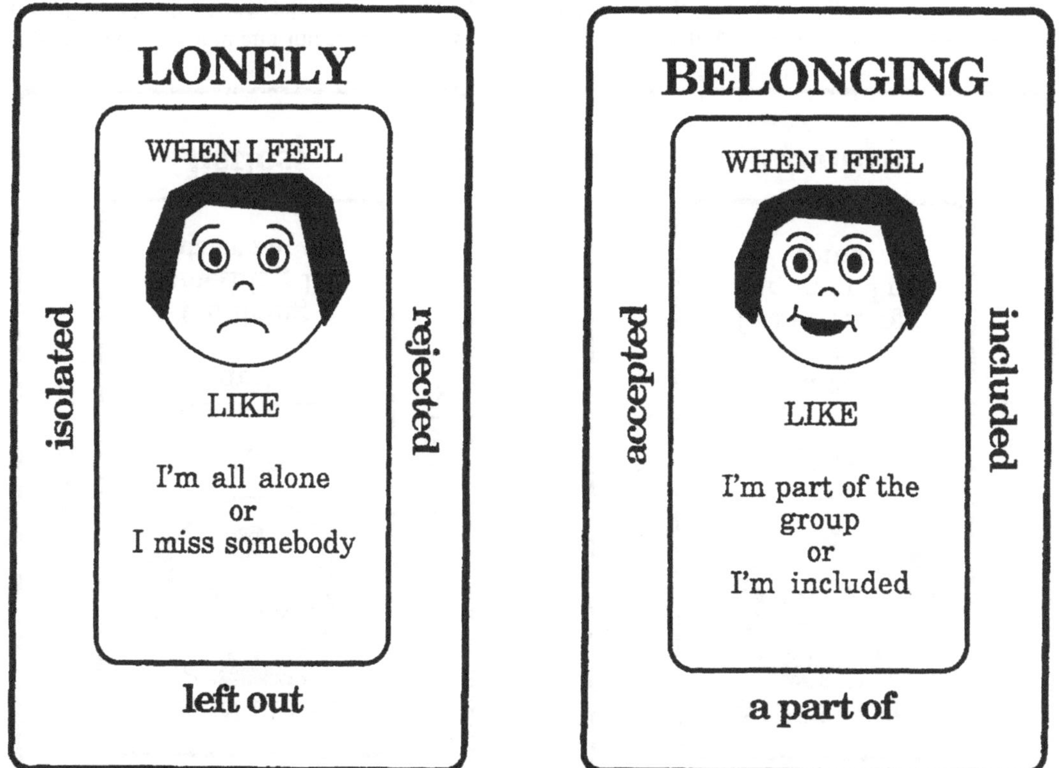

Figure 3.13. Lonely and Belonging feelings cards. Reprinted with permission of The Feelings Factory, Raleigh, NC. Permission is granted to enlarge and photocopy for classroom use.

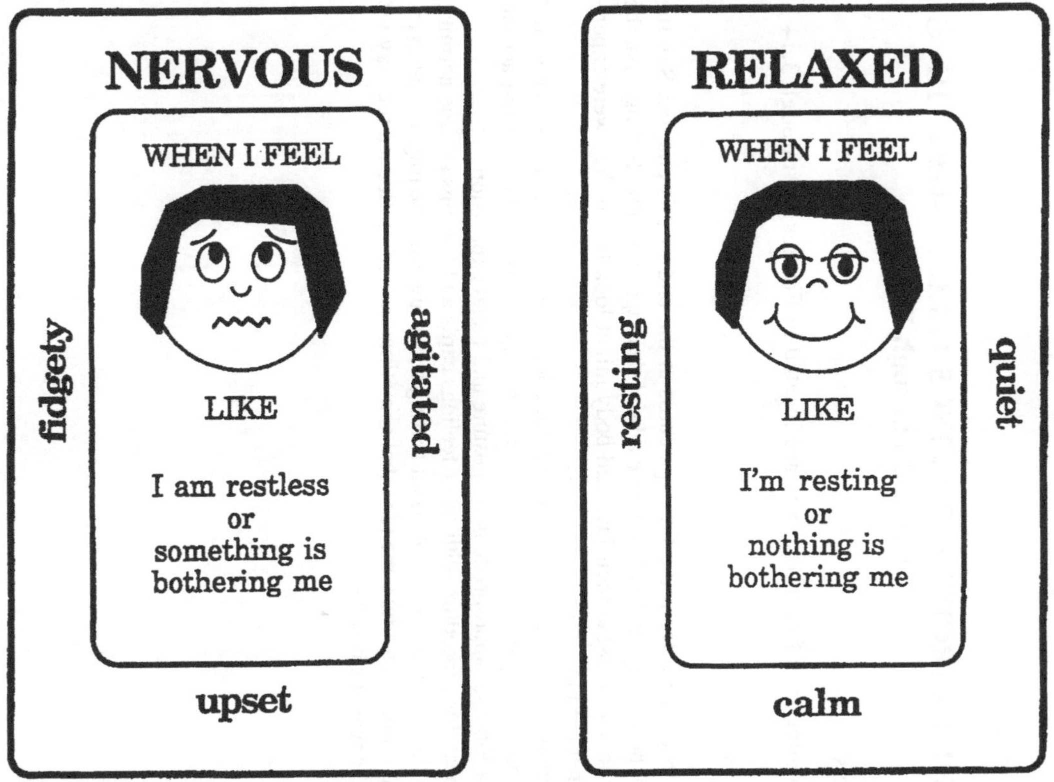

Figure 3.14. Nervous and Relaxed feelings cards. Reprinted with permission of The Feelings Factory, Raleigh, NC. Permission is granted to enlarge and photocopy for classroom use.

STEP I, EXERCISE 5. FEELINGS TELL US SOMETHING (Ages 5 Through 7)

Materials

A photocopy of each feeling card located in Figures 3.7 through 3.14 is needed.

Activity

Choose a card from the feelings cards at the end of this chapter. Say the name of the feeling out loud and give a brief description of that feeling. Ask the children to act out what their face and body might look like if they were experiencing that feeling.

Then ask the children to think of a situation where they could be that would lead to that feeling (e.g., happy, sad, love, hate, etc.). Have the children act out that situation with appropriate body posture and facial expression.

Repeat this procedure with other feelings cards and feelings as time permits.

Tell the children that the pleasant feeling states are ones we might want to repeat, if possible. Introduce the idea that sometimes we can influence the way we feel by the way we behave.

STEP I, EXERCISE 1. FEELINGS HAVE NAMES (Ages 8 Through 11)

Materials

- The feelings listed here are located on cards in Figures 3.7, 3.8, 3.9, and 3.10. Photocopy and separate the cards on the dotted lines so that they can be distributed one at a time to the children. (A culturally sensitive, colorful set of these feelings cards can be purchased through The Feelings Factory, Raleigh, NC, 1-800-858-2264.)

HAPPY	SAD
SATISFIED	ANGRY
PROUD	ASHAMED
SAFE	FRIGHTENED

- Blank paper (one per child)
- Crayons for each child

Activity

Tell the children that sometimes we need words for what we are feeling as changes take place in our lives. We need names for feelings so we can talk about them.

Give each of the children one of the feelings cards. Ask each child to read from his/her card (a) the name of the feeling, (b) the definition of the feeling, and (c) other words that describe the feeling.

Then have the child tell about a situation that children might be experiencing that would lead to their feeling this way. With each separate feeling, allow several children to talk about times when they have felt that way.

If time remains, give each child a Feelings Card and a blank piece of paper to illustrate the word itself in colors and designs that fit the feeling. An example is shown in Figure 3.15.

Suggestion: Integrate the feelings words into the school curricula wherever possible (e.g., as spelling words, in writing assignments, etc.)

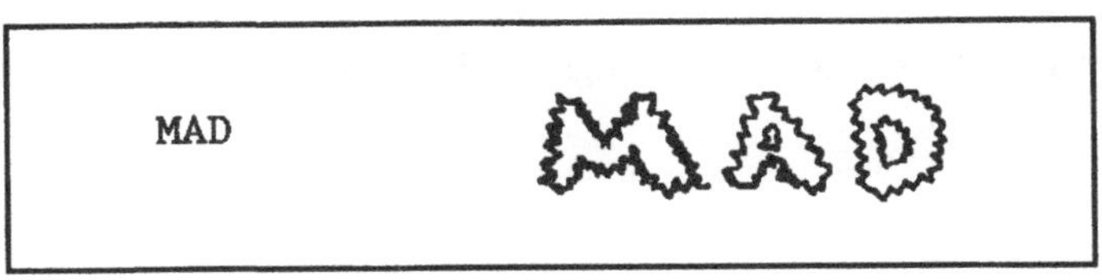

Figure 3.15. Illustration of a feelings word—MAD.

STEP I, EXERCISE 2. FEELINGS HAVE NAMES, Continued (Ages 8 Through 11)

Materials

- The following feelings are located on cards in Figures 3.11, 3.12, 3.13, and 3.14. Photocopy and separate the cards on the dotted lines.

LOVE	HATE
INTERESTED	BORED
BELONGING	LONELY
RELAXED	NERVOUS

- Blank paper (one per child)
- Crayons for each child

Activity

Tell the children that sometimes we need words for what we are feeling as changes take place in our lives. We need names for feelings so we can talk about them.

Give each of the children one of the feelings cards. Ask each child to read from his/her card (a) the name of the feeling, (b) the definition of the feeling, and (c) other words that describe the feeling.

Then have the child tell about a situation that children might be experiencing that would lead to their feeling this way. With each separate feeling, allow several children to talk about times when they have felt that way.

If time remains, give each child a Feelings Card and a blank piece of paper to illustrate the word itself in colors and designs that fit the feeling. An example is shown in Figure 3.16.

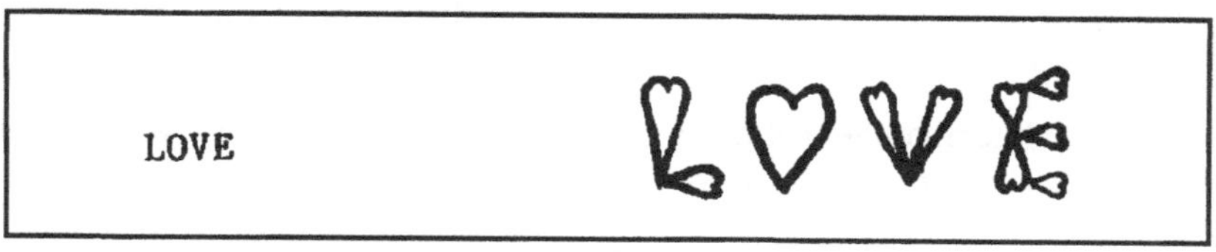

Figure 3.16. Illustration of a feelings word—LOVE.

STEP I, EXERCISE 3. I HAVE FEELINGS (Ages 8 Through 11)

Materials

A photocopy for each child of the *I Have Feelings* fill-in-the-blank sentences (Figure 3.17) is needed.

Activity

Ask the children to read the sentences to themselves on their copy of the page titled *I Have Feelings*. Ask them to read all of the sentences before they write anything in the blanks.

Then have the children read the sentences again and use one of the feelings words to fill in the blank. When completed, ask the children to read the sentences out loud and tell which feeling word they used to complete the sentence. Have the children describe other situations where these same feelings might occur.

I Have Feelings

Use each of the feelings words only once:

HAPPY	PROUD	LOVE	LONELY
SAD	ASHAMED	HATE	BELONGING
ANGRY	SAFE	BORED	NERVOUS
SATISFIED	FRIGHTENED	INTERESTED	RELAXED

1. Imagine your best friend moved. You might feel ____________________.
2. Another word for feeling mad is ____________________.
3. You wanted an ice cream cone all day; then you got to eat one and, when you were done, you might feel ____________________.
4. If you are skating and fall down in front of a group of friends, you might feel ____________________.
5. Imagine you were going for a walk and suddenly an angry-looking dog came running toward you. You might feel ____________________.
6. When things are going just fine, you feel ____________________.
7. Imagine you have completed a tough homework lesson. When you turn it in to the teacher, you may feel ____________________ of yourself.
8. If you feel comfortable, as if nothing can harm you, you feel ____________________.

Figure 3.17. I Have Feelings worksheet. Permission is granted to enlarge and photocopy for classroom use.

STEP I, EXERCISE 4. I HAVE FEELINGS, Continued (Ages 8 Through 11)

Materials

A photocopy for each child of the crossword puzzle (Figure 3.18) is needed.

Activity

Ask the children to complete the crossword puzzle and then share their answers with each other. As they share, have the class describe several circumstances or situations where individuals in the class might feel the given feeling (e.g., bored, lonely, etc.).

Ask the children what they think it means to "Tune in for a change to your inner voice" from the words-to-rhythm jingle, *Reason 'n Rhyme* (Figures 3.2 and 3.3). Help them relate to tuning in to TV channels and that feelings are one important channel to them. If time permits, have children draw a picture of a "feeling face" inside of a television screen.

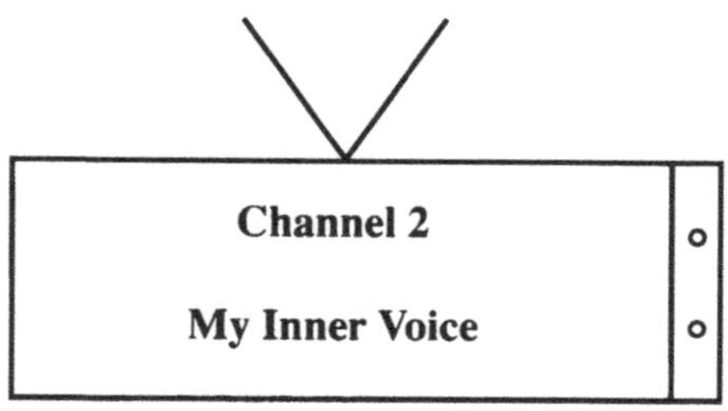

Feelings Crossword Puzzle

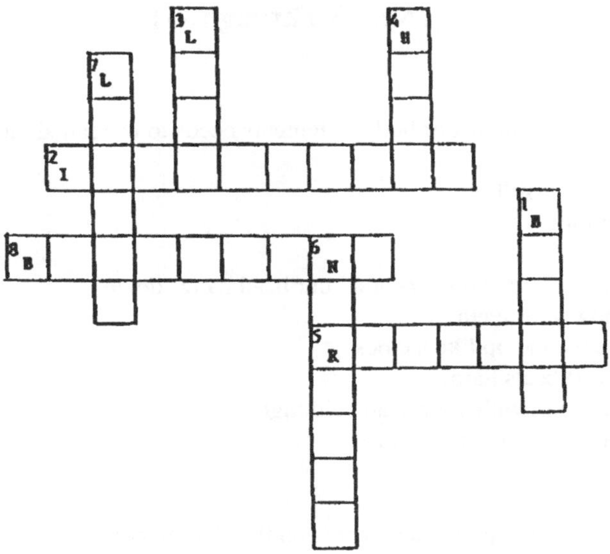

Fill in the boxes above with the correct feelings. Use the following words just once each:

BELONGING	RELAXED	BORED	LOVE
LONELY	NERVOUS	HATE	INTERESTED

1. When I don't have anything interesting to do, I feel ________________.
2. When I am reading a book and want to find out what happened next, I am ________________ in it.
3. If I like my dog very much, I might say that I feel ________________ for the dog.
4. If I really don't like something, I might feel like I ________________ it.
5. Just before I drift off to sleep at night, if I am very still and feel peaceful inside, I feel ________________.
6. When I feel like I have butterflies in my stomach, and I don't feel calm, I am feeling ________________.
7. If I am by myself and wish that my friends were with me, I may be feeling ________________.
8. When I am with a group and feel included I may feel ________________.

Figure 3.18. Feelings Crossword Puzzle. Permission is granted to enlarge and photocopy for classroom use.

STEP I, EXERCISE 5.
BODY CHANGES ACCOMPANY FEELINGS
(Ages 8 Through 11)

Materials

The following list of body statements needs to be read aloud.

You can't sit still.
You go limp.
You cry.
You slump your shoulders and your head hangs down.
You show your teeth.
You are wound up like a clock.
Your heart beats hard.
You stand tall with your head held high.
You have a smile on your face.

Activity

Print the following feelings words on the chalkboard:

NERVOUS	ANGRY
RELAXED	ASHAMED
FRIGHTENED	SAD
PROUD	HAPPY

Tell the children that today they will be talking about how their body changes when their feelings change.

As you read aloud the body statements listed above, ask the children, one at a time, to stand in front of the class and act out what their body would look like if it corresponds to the description you provide with each statement.

Then have the class choose a feelings word from the chalkboard that matches the way the body looks.

Finally, ask a volunteer to describe a situation which might lead to a child feeling this way. Follow with the other statements.

Brainstorm the meaning of the word "Accept." Compare the children's meaning of the word to the definition in the dictionary.

PRACTICAL EXERCISES FOR STEP II—PAUSE

Pause.
Stop and relax!
Free my mind up to guide.

Objective

To help children understand and experience that they can relax and control their body when they are upset or excited, and feel out of control.

The second step in learning to cope is learning how to pause to gain composure and to stop impulsive action. Children can be taught several simple ways to gain composure and control of their own body including deep breathing, counting, imagery, or deep muscle relaxation.

The following body control exercises and scripts have been written with the two age groups in mind—5- through 7-year-olds and 8- through 11-year-olds. In the younger age group, the emphasis in the exercises is placed more on stopping and simple relaxation or body control techniques. In the older age group, more complicated situations and a computer model of relaxation are introduced.

STEP II, EXERCISE 1. I CAN STOP AND RELAX (Ages 5 Through 7)

Introduction

Tell the children that today you will be helping them learn to control and relax their bodies. Ask the children what they think it means to relax. Take several answers.

Problematic Situation

Ask the children to pretend: You will soon go out to play. You feel very excited, and you can't stop your body from moving. Before you can go outside, however, you must concentrate on your class work and finish the assignment.

Step I—Accept

Tell the children that you want their bodies to start moving now. Your hands are moving. Your feet are moving. Your head is moving. Tell them you want them to keep their bodies moving like this until you tell them to stop. Allow the children to move this way for 30 seconds.

Step II—Pause

Then say, "You are feeling very excited. Say to yourself 'I feel excited.' Now, stop moving all the parts of your body one at a time . . . your hands, mouth, feet, head, legs."

Tell the children to close their eyes, to take two deep breaths, and to stay still for a few seconds until you tell them to open their eyes. You'd like for them to stay as still as a turtle resting inside its shell.

Discussion

After the children open their eyes, discuss with them how they felt in both activities (i.e., moving and still). Tell the children that, to gain control of their body, they can stop and relax when they become upset or excited.

Practice

Repeat this exercise several times as an introduction to relaxation and body control. If possible, incorporate it into the children's daily activities by reminding them to use the technique themselves when they feel that their body is out of control. Learning this technique also could be magnified if the teacher or group leader learns to use it and models it for the children.

STEP II, EXERCISE 2. I CAN STOP AND RELAX, Continued (Ages 5 Through 7)

Review

Discuss with the children how relaxing may involve only a few seconds where they pause to gain control of their body. Tell the children that today they are going to learn how to control their body even more on their own.

Remind the children that, in the last exercise, they pretended to be excited about going out to play. Then you told them to stop and take deep breaths. Tell them that this time *they* are going to tell themselves what they are feeling, then stop their body and take a deep breath when you give them a signal to do so. (Make up your own signal—raising your hand, holding up a pencil, etc.).

Problematic Situation

Ask the children to pretend with you: "Someone has just done something to you that made you very angry. Someone took a special cookie, which you had been saving for yourself, off your desk and ate it. You feel angry. Your fists are clenched. Your jaws feel tight. You are gritting your teeth. You feel like you want either to scream, call the person a name, or hit."

Step I—Accept

Now tell the children that, when you give them the signal, you want them to tell themselves silently what they are feeling. (Example: "Now I feel angry.")

Step II—Pause

Next, have the children say to themselves what they can do about this feeling. (Example: "I need to stop and relax." "I need to take a few deep breaths."

Then, after you give them the signal, ask the children to say out loud what they are feeling, to tell themselves to stop and relax, and to take a few deep breaths. If they want to close their eyes, they may.

Discussion

After you have practiced this exercise once or twice with the children, discuss with the children how they felt in both situations (i.e., angry and relaxed). Have the children discuss how relaxing might help them when they become angry with someone.

Practice

Repeat this exercise several times and, if possible, incorporate it into daily activities.

STEP II, EXERCISE 3.
I CAN REMEMBER TO STOP AND RELAX
(Ages 5 Through 7)

Review

Remind the children that, in the last exercise, they were practicing ways to relax and control their body. Tell them that today they are going to practice the steps again and learn to say some things to themselves in their deep breathing.

Problematic Situation

With eyes closed, ask the children to pretend with you: "Your toys are spread all over the house. Your mother or father (or whoever was in charge of you) told you had to pick them all up before you could watch your favorite television program."

Step I—Accept

With eyes open, elicit from the children what they might be feeling (e.g., anger, hopelessness, etc.) and what their body might be doing (e.g., pouting, making faces, etc.).

Step II—Pause

Tell the children to imagine that they are feeling that way now . . . pause . . . Tell them when you give them a signal (i.e., raised hand, etc.), you want them to tell themselves silently: "I feel _____________ (e.g., like pouting, angry, etc.)." "I need to stop, relax, and take a few breaths."

Give them the signal. As they are doing their deep breathing, tell them to blow out the idea that they are going to lose control of their body and do something silly. They are blowing out the "garbage." Then, as they breathe in, ask them to imagine that they are in charge of their body and that they can do something that will help them. Tell them to say silently (i.e., to themselves) as they breathe in, "I can control my body."

Discussion

Discuss with the children their experiences of the relaxation and deep breathing and whether they found it helpful. Ask them to imagine other problematic situations where they could use it.

Practice

Have the children practice this deep breathing several times—breathing out "No more garbage" and breathing in "I can control my body."

Try to choose a time during the daily activities of the children when they are more rowdy or out of control to practice the exercise with them.

STEP II, EXERCISE 4.
I CAN HELP MYSELF BY RELAXING
(Ages 5 Through 7)

Review

Tell the children that today they are going to practice in the same way to identify their feelings, stop, relax, and breathe again so that they can stay in control of their bodies when they become upset. Ask them to think of a pause signal for themselves that would help them stop and relax (e.g., pushing a pretend pause button on hand).

Help the children remember the steps they used in the last session when they pretended to be upset about picking up their toys.

Problematic Situation

Ask them to stand up and pretend with you: "You are getting ready to stand in front of a large audience to recite a poem and sing a song. You want to do a good job but are not sure you can remember the poem. Your hands start to shake, your knees wobble. You feel worried and very nervous. When you're not wobbling, you feel stiff and tight."

Step I—Accept

Tell yourself what you are feeling.

Step II—Pause

Tell yourself to stop all body movements, relax, and take deep breaths, blowing out and saying silently, "No more garbage," breathing in and telling yourself silently, "I can control my body."

Have the children go ahead and wobble, shake, and then get stiff and tight.

Discussion

Discuss with the children their experiences today in practicing this technique. Try to incorporate the technique into their daily activities. Ask the children to think of a favorite place they go at home to relax or a picture they think of in their mind to help them relax.

Practice

Then, tell the children that, as they are ready, practice the steps that you reviewed with them earlier. Talk them through Steps I and II (Accept and Pause). Say them slowly.

STEP II, EXERCISE 5.
I CAN STOP AND RELAX IN TIMES OF TROUBLE
(Ages 5 Through 7)

Introduction and Review

Ask the children to identify times when they or other children they know may become upset, angry, nervous, and lose control of their body. List their examples on the chalkboard or chart paper.

Problematic Situation

Now either (a) have the children vote on the example that is most problematic to them as a group or (b) have each child visualize a situation that is a special problem for them.

Tell the children that you will give them practice in how to control their body when they are in this upsetting situation. If it is a group chosen situation, try to design the specifics of a story, including feelings, body movements, and postures that might go with that situation. If it is a personal situation, help ground the children in the situation by giving them time to close their eyes, visualize where they are, what they are feeling, and what they are doing with their bodies.

Steps I and II—Accept and Pause

Then talk them through the steps cited below. Remind them to think of their own pause signal that helps them remember to stop and relax.

Step I: Tell yourself what you are feeling.
Step II: Tell yourself to stop all body movements, relax, and take deep breaths, blowing out and saying silently, "No more garbage," breathing in and telling yourself silently, "I can control my body."

Discussion

Discuss with the children their problematic situations, whether they were able to visualize them, and the degree of success they had in trying to relax themselves and gain control of their body.

Practice

Tell the children you would like them to practice this exercise the next time they are upset. If feasible, have a separate session for the children to come back and report on their degree of success, with group discussion on ways to improve. Have the children illustrate the pause and relax verse (verse 3) of the words-to-rhythm jingle, *Reason 'n Rhyme* (Figures 3.2 and 3.3).

STEP II, EXERCISE 1. I CAN STOP AND RELAX (Ages 8 Through 11)

Introduction

Tell the children that they will be learning some ways to stop and relax in order to gain control of their body.

Problematic Situation

Tell the children to imagine: "Your brain and body are like a computer. You run on different programs. Your programs are messages you give to yourself or messages others have given to you. Sometimes, when you feel upset, you may have programs that are activated that could lead your mind or body to trouble."

Ask the children to imagine again with you: "You are ready to go outside to play and you are very excited. You are programmed, when you are excited, to move your hands, feet, and head. You can't stop your body from moving."

Step I—Accept

Tell the children to begin moving in that way and to continue moving until you tell them to say, "I am in excitement overload." Have the children say as a group, "I am in excitement overload."

Step II—Pause

Tell the children that you are going to say some things next and that when you say "Relaxation," you want them to stop their bodies from moving and be still (i.e., hands, feet, heads, will all stop moving). Then say, "Relaxation."

Tell the children to close their eyes and when you say "Deep breaths," you want them to take two deep breaths. Then say "Deep breaths."

Discussion

Discuss with the children how it felt to experience the program of excitement overload and how they experienced the new program of learning to stop and relax and take deep breaths in order to get control of their body.

Practice

Repeat this exercise several times as an introduction to help children see themselves as a computer with programs that they can acquire for relaxation and body control. If the teacher or group leader uses and models this technique in daily activities, the children's learning will be enhanced.

STEP II, EXERCISE 2.
I CAN STOP AND RELAX, Continued
(Ages 8 Through 11)

Introduction

Tell the children that today they will be learning more about how to control their own brain and body. You want them to think of themselves again as a computer. They are in charge of this computer. First they will listen to their body's program when they feel angry. Then they will learn how to reprogram themselves with new programs that will help them relax and control their bodies.

Problematic Situation

Ask the children to imagine with you: "You are going to play soccer at recess. The teacher says that the children who take the ball outside get to be team captains for the day. You have the ball and take it outside when suddenly a bully from an older class comes over and grabs the ball, saying, 'Thanks for the ball, kid.' As he walks away with it, you start to feel angry. Your fists are clenched, and your jaws feel tight. You are gritting your teeth and you feel like you want to scream or run after the bully and hit him."

Steps I and II—Accept and Pause

Tell the children that you want them to tighten their jaws, grit their teeth, clench their fists, and feel the anger inside them. Now, when you give them a signal (e.g., raise you finger, clap your hand, etc.), you want them to tell themselves how they feel. Next, they should remind themselves to pause and relax.

Step I—Accept: "I feel angry. Anger overload."
Step II—Pause: "Stop body movement. Relax."

Write these steps on the chalkboard. Give the signal. Allow children time to go through the steps.

Now tell the children to say quietly to themselves, "Deep breaths," and to go ahead and take several deep breaths.

Discussion

Discuss with the children how it felt to experience the program of anger overload and how they experienced the new program of learning to stop and relax in order to gain control of their body.

Practice

Repeat this exercise several times to help children see themselves as computers with programs that they can acquire for relaxation and body control.

STEP II, EXERCISE 3.
I CAN REMEMBER TO STOP AND RELAX
(Ages 8 Through 11)

Introduction and Review

Write the following on the chalkboard:

I feel ____________. (Step I—Accept)
Stop body movement. Relax and take deep breaths. (Step II—Pause)

Tell the children that you will describe a situation and, when you give them a signal, you want them to go through the above two steps.

Problematic Situation

Ask the children to imagine: "You are getting ready to go out to play with friends. Your friends have not been around for several days, and you've been looking forward to playing with them. They have to be home in a couple of hours for supper. As you're just getting ready to walk out the door, your mother or father (or whoever is in charge of you) says, 'You have to stay in now until you wash the dishes, pick up your toys throughout the house, and clean your room.' You expect that this will take at least an hour, and you know that your friends will be gone by then."

Elicit from the children what they might be feeling (e.g., anger, frustration, hopelessness, etc.). With each feeling mentioned, have the children describe what their body might be doing. Have the children imagine that they're feeling that way now and that each one of them may be feeling something different. Tell them: "Remember, you have to stay in, your friends are gone, you don't want to miss your play time."

Steps I and II—Accept and Pause

Tell the children that when you give them a signal, you want them to go through the steps listed on the chalkboard. Give the signal. As the children begin the deep breathing step, tell them, "When you breathe out, say to yourself, 'No more garbage.' When you breathe in, say to yourself, 'I can control my body.'"

Discussion

Discuss with the children their experiences of the relaxation and deep breathing. Ask them to imagine other circumstances where they could use it. Brainstorm the meaning of relaxation and its opposites. Talk about obstacles to stopping and relaxing.

Practice

Practice this exercise when the children are rowdy or out of control.

STEP II, EXERCISE 4.
I CAN HELP MYSELF BY RELAXING
(Ages 8 Through 11)

Introduction and Review

Review with the children the four coping steps and emphasize how stopping and relaxing is an important second step when they become upset. Help the children remember the steps they used in the last session when they pretended to be upset about not getting to play with their friends. Write the steps on the chalkboard again:

I feel ____________ . (Step I—Accept)
Stop body movement. Relax and take deep breaths. (Step II—Pause)
  Breathe out and say to yourself, "No more garbage."
  Breathe in and say to yourself, "I can control my body."

Tell the children that they are going to practice these steps to gain control of their bodies.

Problematic Situation

Ask the children to stand up and walk in place. Say to them: "You are walking up to your front door with a note from your teacher. The note says you have not done your work today and have caused trouble for other children in the classroom. You open the front door. Your mother or father (or whoever is in charge of you) goes to answer the telephone just about the time the teacher had said she would call to discuss these problems with them. As the phone rings, your hands start to shake, your knees wobble, you feel stiff, tight, and sweaty."

Steps I and II—Accept and Pause

Ask the children to imagine how they might be feeling, but to keep it to themselves. Then have the children go through the steps listed on the chalkboard.

Discussion

After everyone has finished, process with the children what they were feeling and then how it felt to relax.

Practice

Try to incorporate this technique into daily practice whenever possible.

STEP II, EXERCISE 5.
I CAN STOP AND RELAX IN TIMES OF TROUBLE
(Ages 8 Through 11)

Introduction

Ask the children to identify times when they or other children they know may become upset, angry, nervous, and lose control of their body.

Problematic Situation

List their examples on the chalkboard or chart paper. Now either (a) have the children vote on the example that is most problematic to them as a group or (b) have each child visualize a situation that is especially problematic to him/her.

Tell the children that you are going to give them practice in how to control their body when they're in this upsetting situation. If it is a group chosen situation, try to design the specifics of a story, including feelings, body movements and postures that might go with that situation. If it is a personal situation, help ground the children in the situation by giving them time to close their eyes, visualize where they are, what they are feeling, and what they are doing with their bodies.

Steps I and II—Accept and Pause

Put the steps listed below on the chalkboard. Then talk the children through the steps of how they can stop, relax, and gain control of their body.

I feel ______________. (Step I—Accept)
Stop body movement. Relaxation and take deep breaths. (Step II—Pause)
  Breathe out and say to yourself, "No more garbage."
  Breathe in and say to yourself, "I can control my body."

Discussion

Discuss with the children their problematic situations, whether they were able to visualize them, and the degree of success they had in trying to relax themselves and gain control of their body.

Practice

Tell the children you would like them to practice this exercise the next time they are upset. Have them report on their success and problems.

PRACTICAL EXERCISES FOR STEP III—THINK

Think.
Go and think!
I have choices to make.

Objective

To help children understand and experience their own ability to think constructively. This includes considering options for actions that are not harmful to themselves or others.

Thinking follows body control or composure as the third step in learning to cope. Thinking involves generating options for action, deciding which of these options could help, and creating a plan for action.

When children think of options for action, they usually are not selective. Some of the options they think of would have harmful consequences if pursued. Other options are helpful. Still others may appear to contain both helpful and harmful elements. While children are brainstorming, all options should be considered as viable choices for action because we want to encourage the process of thinking. The idea is to accept all the children's suggestions as possible choices, but to help them think through to the consequences of their actions.

Exercises to build skills in thinking constructively are provided for the two age groups—5- through 7-year-olds and 8- through 11-year-olds.

STEP III, EXERCISE 1. I CAN THINK AND MAKE GOOD CHOICES (Ages 5 Through 7)

Introduction

Tell the children that you will be talking with them today about thinking. Thinking is about using our brain, coming up with ideas, and making choices that are helpful. Thinking helps us find ways to help ourselves when we become upset.

Problematic Situation

From the story, *Tom and Jeri Learn to Cope* (Introductory Exercise 1), review the situation when Tom suggests playing soccer and then calls Jeri names because he is disappointed that she will not play. Ask the children to imagine: "Tom said to you, 'Baby, baby, you are a baby. You can't kick the ball. That's why you don't want to play.' What might you be feeling?"

Steps I and II—Accept and Pause

Write Steps I and II on the chalkboard, and then lead the children through both until they are relaxed.

Tell yourself what you are feeling. (Step I—Accept)
Tell yourself to stop all body movement, relax, and take deep breaths.
(Step II—Pause)
Breathe out and say to yourself, "No more garbage."
Breathe in and say to yourself, "I can control my body."

Step III—Think

As children become relaxed, ask them to think internally, in a relaxed state, of all the possible things Jeri could do when she hears Tom say these things.

Allow the children to tell you what options they thought about. List Jeri's options on the chalkboard. Be sure to include even silly options or ideas from the children.

Discussion

Discuss what might occur with each of the options.

Practice

Finally, using the relaxation technique that they have learned, have the children relax again and think about which one of these choices would be least harmful to Jeri and others. Ask the class to vote on the one choice they believe is least harmful to Jeri or others.

Congratulate the class on thinking. Tell them that brainstorming, thinking of options, and looking ahead is what thinking is all about.

STEP III, EXERCISE 2.
I CAN THINK OF WAYS TO HELP MYSELF
(Ages 5 Through 7)

Introduction

Remind the children that, several sessions ago, they imagined with you that someone took a special cookie off their desk and ate it. They felt very angry.

Problematic Situation

Ask the children to imagine: "You are there again right now. Your fists are clenched, your jaws are tight, and you're gritting your teeth. You feel like you want to scream, call names, or hit."

Steps I, II, and III—Accept, Pause, and Think

Now ask the children to remember the steps that help them understand what they are feeling and gain body control. Write these steps on the chalkboard. Then go through each step with the children.

Tell yourself what you are feeling. (Step I—Accept)
Tell yourself to stop all body movement, relax, and take deep breaths. (Step II—Pause)
  Breathe out and say to yourself, "No more garbage."
  Breathe in and say to yourself, "I can control my body."
Tell yourself to think. Think of ways to help yourself. (Step III—Think)

As children become relaxed, ask them to remain relaxed and think of all the possible things they could do in this situation. Ask them to tell you what options they thought of. Place the options on the chalkboard. Include all options, even apparently "silly ones."

Discussion

Discuss what might occur with each option. Ask the children to relax for a moment and think again about which option would be most helpful, keeping in mind respect for themselves and the other person. Then ask the class to vote on which option they think is most helpful and why.

Practice

Discuss how the whole process followed in this lesson could be helpful in other situations when they might become angry. Have the children describe the circumstance and model the accepting, pausing, thinking steps in those circumstances.

STEP III, EXERCISE 3.
I CAN THINK OF WAYS TO HELP MYSELF WHEN I AM FEELING UPSET
(Ages 5 Through 7)

Introduction and Problematic Situation

Remind the children that, several sessions ago, you asked them to imagine with you that their toys were spread all over the house and that they had to pick them up before they could watch their favorite TV program. You want them to go back into that situation now and imagine with you what they are thinking and feeling.

Steps I, II, and III—Accept, Pause, and Think

Now ask the children to remember the steps that help them understand what they are feeling and gain body control. Write these steps on the chalkboard. Then go through each step with the children.

Tell yourself what you are feeling. (Step I—Accept)
Tell yourself to stop all body movement, relax, and take deep breaths. (Step II—Pause)
  Breathe out and say to yourself, "No more garbage."
  Breathe in and say to yourself, "I can control my body."
Tell yourself to think. Think of ways to help yourself. (Step III—Think)

As children become relaxed, ask them to remain relaxed and think of all the possible things they could do in this situation. Ask them to tell you what options they thought of. Place the options on the chalkboard. Include all options, even apparently "silly ones."

Discussion

Discuss what might occur with each option. Ask the children to relax for a moment and think again about which option would be most helpful, keeping in mind respect for themselves and the other people involved. Then ask the class to vote on which option they think is most helpful and why.

Practice

Discuss how the whole process followed in this lesson could be helpful in other situations when they might become angry. Have the children describe the circumstance and model the accepting, pausing, thinking steps in those circumstances.

STEP III, EXERCISE 4. I CAN THINK OF WAYS TO HELP MYSELF WHEN I AM FEELING ANXIOUS OR NERVOUS (Ages 5 Through 7)

Introduction and Problematic Situation

Remind the children that, several sessions ago, you asked them to imagine with you that they are getting ready to stand in front of a large audience and recite a poem and sing a song. Tell them: "You want to do a good job but are not sure you can remember the poem. Your hands start to shake and your knees wobble. You feel worried and very nervous. When you're not wobbling, you feel stiff and tight." Have the children get back into the imagined situation and wobble and shake, then get stiff and tight.

Steps I, II, and III—Accept, Pause, and Think

Now ask the children to remember the steps that help them understand what they are feeling and gain body control. Write these steps on the chalkboard. Then go through each step with the children.

Tell yourself what you are feeling. (Step I—Accept)
Tell yourself to stop all body movement, relax, and take deep breaths. (Step II—Pause)
  Breathe out and say to yourself, "No more garbage."
  Breathe in and say to yourself, "I can control my body."
Tell yourself to think. Think of ways to help yourself. (Step III—Think)

As children become relaxed, ask them to remain relaxed and think of all the possible things they could do in this situation. Ask them to tell you what options they thought of. Place the options on the chalkboard. Include all options, even apparently "silly ones."

Discussion

Discuss what might occur with each option. Ask the children to relax for a moment and think again about which option would be most helpful, keeping in mind respect for themselves. Then ask the class to vote on which option they think is most helpful and why.

Practice

Discuss how the whole process followed in this lesson could be helpful in other situations when they might become angry. Have the children describe the circumstance and model the accepting, pausing, thinking steps in those circumstances.

STEP III, EXERCISE 5. I CAN THINK OF WAYS TO HELP MYSELF IN TIMES OF TROUBLE (Ages 5 Through 7)

Introduction and Problematic Situation

Tell the children to recall a time when they became upset, angry, or other emotion. Tell them that you are going to give them practice in how to control their body when they are in this upsetting situation. Help ground the children in the situation by giving them time to close their eyes, visualize where they are, what they are feeling, and what they are doing with their bodies.

Steps I, II, and III—Accept, Pause, and Think

Now ask the children to remember the steps that help them understand what they are feeling and gain body control. Write these steps on the chalkboard. Then go through each step with the children.

Tell yourself what you are feeling. (Step I—Accept)
Tell yourself to stop all body movement, relax, and take deep breaths. (Step II—Pause)
  Breathe out and say to yourself, "No more garbage."
  Breathe in and say to yourself, "I can control my body."
Tell yourself to think. Think of ways to help yourself. (Step III—Think)

Ask for one or two children to volunteer to tell their situation out loud so that the class can help think of options. Place the options on the chalkboard. Include all options, even apparently "silly ones."

Discussion

Discuss what might occur with each option. Ask the children to relax for a moment and think again about which option would be most helpful. Then ask the class to vote on which option they think is most helpful and why.

Practice

Have the children role-play two or three of the situations and how they would identify feelings (accept), relax (pause), and think of an option (think) that could help them without hurting others.

STEP III, EXERCISE 1. I CAN MAKE GOOD CHOICES WHEN I FEEL EXCITED (Ages 8 Through 11)

Introduction and Problematic Situation

Ask the children to remember the time when they imagined that they were getting ready to go outside to play and they were very excited. Like a computer, they were *programmed* when they were excited to move their hands, feet, and head. They could not stop their bodies from moving. Ask them to pretend they are in that situation again. Their *program* of moving hands and feet is *switched on*.

Steps I, II, and III—Accept, Pause, and Think

Help the children go through the following steps:

I feel ____________. (Step I—Accept)
Stop body movement. Relax and take deep breaths. (Step II—Pause)
  Breathe out and say to yourself, "No more garbage."
  Breathe in and say to yourself, "I can control my body."
Think of program options. (Step III—Think)

As the children become relaxed, ask them to begin thinking about all the possible things they could do (i.e., all the *program options*) at this time.

Ask the children to tell you all the program options they thought of for action in this situation. Tell them you want to hear all the possibilities, even the silly ones. Write the following four headings on the chalkboard: "Situation and Feelings," "Program Options," "Consequences," and "Helpful or Harmful."

After describing and writing the *situation and feelings*, list the children's suggestions under *program options*. Engage the class in deciding the *consequences* and whether the options are *helpful or harmful*. Ask the class to vote on which option could be most helpful to them. An example is as follows:

Situation and Feelings	*Program Options*	*Consequences*	*Helpful or Harmful*
Going out to play; excitement, body moving out of control	Deep breathing to stay relaxed	Relaxation and body control	Helpful
	Tell yourself to stop moving	Body control	Helpful
	Let your body go wild	Trouble	Harmful
	Scream	More trouble	Harmful

Discussion

Discuss with the children how their brain and body are like a computer. The children themselves are the computer operators. They can program themselves with options.

Practice

Talk through the following steps with the children.

I feel _____________ . (Step I—Accept)
Stop body movement. Relaxation and take deep breaths. (Step II—Pause)
  Breathe out and say to yourself, "No more garbage."
  Breathe in and say to yourself, "I can control my body."
Think of program options. (Step III—Think)

STEP III, EXERCISE 2. I CAN MAKE GOOD CHOICES WHEN I FEEL ANGRY (Ages 8 Through 11)

Introduction and Problematic Situation

Ask the children to remember when they imagined they were made the team captain to play soccer. Then, a bully from an older class grabbed the ball from them and said, "Thanks for the ball, kid," and walked away.

Try to imagine yourself back there now: "You're very angry. Your fists are clenched. Your jaw is tight. You're gritting your teeth. You feel like you want to scream, run after the bully, and hit him. Your program of anger overload is switched on."

Steps I, II, and III—Accept, Pause, and Think

Help the children go through the following steps:

I feel ____________ . (Step I—Accept)
Stop body movement. Relax and take deep breaths. (Step II—Pause)
  Breathe out and say to yourself, "No more garbage."
  Breathe in and say to yourself, "I can control my body."
Think of program options. (Step III—Think)

As the children become relaxed, ask them to begin thinking about all the possible things they could do (i.e., all the *program options*) at this time.

Ask the children to tell you all the program options they thought of for action in this situation. Tell them you want to hear all the possibilities, even the silly ones. Write the following four headings on the chalkboard: "Situation and Feelings," "Program Options," "Consequences," and "Helpful or Harmful."

After describing and writing the *situation and feelings* under the heading, list the children's suggestions under *program options*. Engage the class in deciding the *consequences* and whether the options are *helpful or harmful*. Ask the class to vote on which option could be most helpful to them.

Practice

Talk through Steps I, II, and III with the children.

STEP III, EXERCISE 3. I CAN MAKE GOOD CHOICES WHEN I FEEL FRUSTRATED AND UPSET (Ages 8 Through 11)

Introduction and Problem Situation

Ask the children to remember when they imagined that they were not allowed to play with their friends. Someone had said to them, "You have to stay in until you wash the dishes, pick up your toys, and clean your room." You knew your friends would be gone when you were finished. You wanted so much to play with your friends that day.

Ask the children to try to imagine themselves back there now. "Remember, you have to stay in. Your friends are leaving. You don't want to miss your playtime. Your mind and your body are both upset. Your program of anger, or frustration, or sadness overload is switched on."

Steps I, II, and III—Accept, Pause, and Think

Help the children go through the following steps:

I feel ____________ . (Step I—Accept)
Stop body movement. Relax and take deep breaths. (Step II—Pause)
  Breathe out and say to yourself, "No more garbage."
  Breathe in and say to yourself, "I can control my body."
Think of program options. (Step III—Think)

As the children become relaxed, ask them to begin thinking about all the possible things they could do (i.e., all the *program options*) at this time.

Ask the children to tell you all the program options they thought of for action in this situation. Tell them you want to hear all the possibilities, even the silly ones. Write the following four headings on the chalkboard: "Situation and Feelings," "Program Options," "Consequences," and "Helpful or Harmful."

After describing and writing the *situation and feelings* under the heading, list the children's suggestions under *program options*. Engage the class in deciding the *consequences* and whether the options are *helpful or harmful*. Ask the class to vote on which option could be most helpful to them.

Practice

Talk through Steps I, II, and III with the children.

STEP III, EXERCISE 4.
I CAN THINK AND MAKE GOOD CHOICES WHEN I FEEL EMBARRASSED AND ANXIOUS
(Ages 8 Through 11)

Introduction and Problematic Situation

Ask the children to stand up. Then ask the children to remember when they imagined they walked up to the front door with a note from their teacher saying that they had caused trouble that day in school.

Ask the children to try to imagine themselves back there now: "You're walking up to the front door (have the children walk in place). The phone is ringing with the teacher on the other end. Your hands start to shake. Your knees wobble. You feel stiff, tight, and sweaty. Your program of anxiety or frustration overload is switched on."

Steps I, II, and III—Accept, Pause, and Think

Help the children go through the following steps:

I feel ____________. (Step I—Accept)
Stop body movement. Relax and take deep breaths. (Step II—Pause)
  Breathe out and say to yourself, "No more garbage."
  Breathe in and say to yourself, "I can control my body."
Think of program options. (Step III—Think)

As the children become relaxed, ask them to begin thinking about all the possible things they could do (i.e., all the *program options*) at this time.

Ask the children to tell you all the program options they thought of for action in this situation. Tell them you want to hear all the possibilities, even the silly ones. Write the following four headings on the chalkboard: "Situation and Feelings," "Program Options," "Consequences," and "Helpful or Harmful."

After describing and writing the *situation and feelings* under the heading, list the children's suggestions under *program options*. Engage the class in deciding the *consequences* and whether the options are *helpful or harmful*. Ask the class to vote on which option could be most helpful to them.

Practice

Talk through the Steps I, II, and III with the children.

STEP III, EXERCISE 5. I CAN THINK IN TIMES OF TROUBLE (Ages 8 Through 11)

Introduction and Problematic Situation

Ask the children to think about a situation when they felt particularly uncomfortable or upset. They may have been angry, nervous, sad, frightened, or had some other unpleasant feeling.

Give the children a few moments to think about that situation. Then tell them to try to remember where they were, who was with them, what they were seeing, smelling, and doing. Allow them a few more minutes to think. Remind them to try to touch their feelings and to think about the feeling that is the strongest for them.

Ask for a volunteer to share his/her story. Apply the rest of this exercise to the volunteer's situation and then to as many children's situations as time allows.

Steps I, II, and III—Accept, Pause, and Think

Ask the children to tell you all the program options they thought of for action in this situation. Tell them you want to hear all the possibilities, even the silly ones. Write the following four headings on the chalkboard: "Situation and Feelings," "Program Options," "Consequences," and "Helpful or Harmful."

After describing and writing the *situation and feelings* under the heading, list the children's suggestions under *program options*. Engage the class in deciding the *consequences* and whether the options are *helpful or harmful*. Ask the class to vote on which option could be most helpful to them.

PRACTICAL EXERCISES FOR STEP IV—DO

Do.
Go and take action!
Put my best choice in place.

Objective

To help children understand the importance of taking positive actions after reviewing their options in difficult situations. Action should be helpful to the self and not harmful to others.

A well-thought-out plan remains just that—a plan—until it is acted upon. Even the best of plans can not help unless action follows.

When encouraging children to act on the best choice for now, it is important to look at the consequences of all the choices so that the children have a better chance of choosing one that will work. This best choice is not harmful to the self or others. Exercises that emphasize doing (action) are provided for both age groups—5- through 7-year-olds and 8- through 11-year-olds.

STEP IV, EXERCISE 1.
I CAN ACT ON MY BEST CHOICE
(Ages 5 Through 7)

Introduction

Tell the class that today they will be working on ways to integrate and practice all four of the coping steps together.

Procedure

For the following vignette, follow the procedure listed here:

1. Read the vignette to the children.
2. Choose actors from the class to play different roles in the story.
3. Act out the story. Read the vignette again, this time prompting the children to act out the roles of the story and any words they might say to each other.
4. Begin Coping Steps I and II—Accept and Pause. Have the actors model the first two steps of the coping model by saying "I am feeling ______________ " and then stopping all body movement, relaxing, and taking deep breaths.
5. Begin Coping Step III—Think. Have the whole class describe the main characters' feelings, options, whether they are helpful or harmful, and best choices. Be sure to describe the feelings, options, etc. of all the actors. On the chalkboard, record the children's comments in four columns: "Feelings," "Options," "Helpful or Harmful," and "Choices."
6. Begin Coping Step IV—Do. Have the actor(s) act out one or more of the *best choices* as determined by the group for one of the actors. Then if a second actor is utilized, proceed with acting out the best choices for the second actor with that actor taking the initiative in the role-play. When completed, two separate best choices could be acted out.

Vignette—"I'm Not Very Good"

Tom and his friends were playing tag outside at recess. Butch and Jeri were really fast. They kept tagging Tom and making him it. It began to seem like Tom was always it. He was not very fast and had difficulty trying to catch them before they ran and touched base. After a while, they began to laugh at Tom and whispered to one another about how slow he was and that he was not very good at the game. Tom knew they were making fun of him.

STEP IV, EXERCISE 2. I CAN ACT ON MY BEST CHOICE, Continued (Ages 5 Through 7)

Introduction

Tell the class that today they will be working on ways to integrate and practice all four of the coping steps together.

Procedure

For the following vignette, follow the procedure listed here:

1. Read the vignette to the children.
2. Choose actors from the class to play different roles in the story.
3. Act out the story. Read the vignette again, this time prompting the children to act out the roles of the story and any words they might say to each other.
4. Begin Coping Steps I and II—Accept and Pause. Have the actors model the first two steps of the coping model by saying "I am feeling ____________ " and then stopping all body movement, relaxing, and taking deep breaths.
5. Begin Coping Step III—Think. Have the whole class describe the main characters' feelings, options, whether they are helpful or harmful, and best choices. Be sure to describe the feelings, options, etc. of all the actors. On the chalkboard, record the children's comments in four columns: "Feelings," "Options," "Helpful or Harmful," and "Choices."
6. Begin Coping Step IV—Do. Have the actor(s) act out one or more of the *best choices* as determined by the group for one of the actors. Then if a second actor is utilized, proceed with acting out the best choices for the second actor with that actor taking the initiative in the role-play. When completed, two separate best choices could be acted out.

Vignette—"No One to Play with"

The teacher announced to the class that it was free time and that each person could choose a game to play. Everyone in the class started to get into groups to play with different things. Some were playing with the kitchen set, some with cars and trucks, and some with blocks. Felicia noticed that Meagan, the new child, was not playing with anyone. She was still sitting at her desk all by herself. Felicia asked her friends, "Why don't we ask the new girl if she wants to play with us? She is all by herself and isn't playing anything." Felicia's friends did not answer. They just kept playing in the kitchen with the pans and dolls.

STEP IV, EXERCISE 3.
I CAN ACT ON MY BEST CHOICE, Continued
(Ages 5 Through 7)

Introduction

Tell the class that today they will be working on ways to integrate and practice all four of the coping steps together.

Procedure

For the following vignette, follow the procedure listed here:

1. Read the vignette to the children.
2. Choose actors from the class to play different roles in the story.
3. Act out the story. Read the vignette again, this time prompting the children to act out the roles of the story and any words they might say to each other.
4. Begin Coping Steps I and II—Accept and Pause. Have the actors model the first two steps of the coping model by saying "I am feeling ____________ " and then stopping all body movement, relaxing, and taking deep breaths.
5. Begin Coping Step III—Think. Have the whole class describe the main characters' feelings, options, whether they are helpful or harmful, and best choices. Be sure to describe the feelings, options, etc. of all the actors. On the chalkboard, record the children's comments in four columns: "Feelings," "Options," "Helpful or Harmful," and "Choices."
6. Begin Coping Step IV—Do. Have the actor(s) act out one or more of the *best choices* as determined by the group for one of the actors. Then if a second actor is utilized, proceed with acting out the best choices for the second actor with that actor taking the initiative in the role-play. When completed, two separate best choices could be acted out.

Vignette—"Tattler"

Billy and his friends were playing on the swings at recess. Everyone had been told by their teacher to take turns on the playground. Each child was taking a turn and sharing the swings. It was now Billy's turn to get on the swing, but another child in his class would not get off of the swing to let Billy have a turn. Billy told Johnny, "It's my turn now. You already have had a chance to swing. We are supposed to share." Johnny told Billy, "I'm not ready to stop swinging. I just got on the swing." Billy knew that Johnny's turn was up, so he went to tell his teacher that Johnny would not take turns and share. His teacher did not tell him that he was right and that Johnny needed to get off the swing. Instead she asked Billy if he was tattling and told him that he was not to be telling on his classmates.

STEP IV, EXERCISE 4. I CAN ACT ON MY BEST CHOICE, Continued (Ages 5 Through 7)

Introduction

Tell the class that today they will be working on ways to integrate and practice all four of the coping steps together.

Procedure

For the following vignette, follow the procedure listed here:

1. Read the vignette to the children.
2. Choose actors from the class to play different roles in the story.
3. Act out the story. Read the vignette again, this time prompting the children to act out the roles of the story and any words they might say to each other.
4. Begin Coping Steps I and II—Accept and Pause. Have the actors model the first two steps of the coping model by saying "I am feeling ____________ " and then stopping all body movement, relaxing, and taking deep breaths.
5. Begin Coping Step III—Think. Have the whole class describe the main characters' feelings, options, whether they are helpful or harmful, and best choices. Be sure to describe the feelings, options, etc. of all the actors. On the chalkboard, record the children's comments in four columns: "Feelings," "Options," "Helpful or Harmful," and "Choices."
6. Begin Coping Step IV—Do. Have the actor(s) act out one or more of the *best choices* as determined by the group for one of the actors. Then if a second actor is utilized, proceed with acting out the best choices for the second actor with that actor taking the initiative in the role-play. When completed, two separate best choices could be acted out.

Vignette—"Taking Turns"

One day Sarah's class was discussing a story they had read in class. Sarah raised her hand to answer her teacher's question, but everyone kept blurting out the answers. No one waited for the teacher to call on them to answer. Sarah tried to get the teacher to notice her, but she was not called on.

STEP IV, EXERCISE 5. I CAN ACT ON MY BEST CHOICE, Continued (Ages 5 Through 7)

Introduction

Tell the class that today they will be working on ways to integrate and practice all four of the coping steps together.

Procedure

For the following vignette, follow the procedure listed here:

1. Read the vignette to the children.
2. Choose actors from the class to play different roles in the story.
3. Act out the story. Read the vignette again, this time prompting the children to act out the roles of the story and any words they might say to each other.
4. Begin Coping Steps I and II—Accept and Pause. Have the actors model the first two steps of the coping model by saying "I am feeling ______" and then stopping all body movement, relaxing, and taking deep breaths.
5. Begin Coping Step III—Think. Have the whole class describe the main characters' feelings, options, whether they are helpful or harmful, and best choices. Be sure to describe the feelings, options, etc. of all the actors. On the chalkboard, record the children's comments in four columns: "Feelings," "Options," "Helpful or Harmful," and "Choices."
6. Begin Coping Step IV—Do. Have the actor(s) act out one or more of the *best choices* as determined by the group for one of the actors. Then if a second actor is utilized, proceed with acting out the best choices for the second actor with that actor taking the initiative in the role-play. When completed, two separate best choices could be acted out.

Vignette—"Keeping Your Hands and Feet to Yourself"

Everyone was sitting on the floor in a circle listening to their teacher read them a story. Ted's friend Barry started pushing him and telling him to move over. Ted turned to Barry and said, "No, this is my spot!" Ted and Barry began arguing and pushing one another. They stopped after they heard their teacher call out their names.

STEP IV, EXERCISE 1.
I CAN ACT ON MY BEST CHOICE
(Ages 8 Through 11)

Introduction

Tell the class that today they will be working on ways to integrate and practice all four of the coping steps together.

Procedure

Select the following children to lead the class in the vignette role-play:

Reader: The reader will read the vignette.
Actors: The actors will act out the different roles in the story.
Teacher: You will prompt the actors in the vignette in their roles and any words they might say to each other.
Coach: The coach will instruct the actors in the first two steps of the coping model by prompting them so that they say what they're feeling and then relax and take deep breaths.
Mediator: The mediator will lead the class in brainstorming possible options for the main actor(s) and will help the class determine best choices that are non-violent and are respectful to the self and others.
Director: The director is responsible for leading the actor(s) in acting out the best choice, as determined by the group.

Have the reader proceed to read the vignette to the other children. Have the reader read the vignette again. Prompt the children to act out the roles of the story and any words they might say to each other.

The coach will begin Coping Steps I and II. Have the actors model the first two steps of the coping model by saying I am feeling " ______________ " and then stopping and taking deep breaths and relaxing.

The mediator will begin Coping Step III. Have the whole class describe the main characters' options and best choices, making sure to describe the feelings, options, etc. of all the actors. Record children's descriptions on the chalkboard in four columns: "Feelings," "Options," "Helpful or Harmful," and "Best Choices."

The director will begin Coping Step IV, directing the actor(s) to act out (do) one or more of the best choices as determined by the group (best choices do not harm oneself or other people). If a second actor is utilized, proceed with acting out the best choices for the second actor, with that actor taking the initiative in the role-play. When completed, two or more separate best choices could be acted out.

Vignette—"Psst! Tell Me the Answer."

You are sitting in class taking a test when the person behind you sticks you in the back with his pencil and says, "Psst, what's the answer to #5?" The teacher hears something and looks up just in time to see you glancing back at your neighbor to see what stuck you. He assumes you are trying to cheat on the test and takes your paper telling you that you will receive an F on the test.

STEP IV, EXERCISE 2.
I CAN ACT ON MY BEST CHOICE, Continued
(Ages 8 Through 11)

Introduction

Tell the class that today they will be working on ways to integrate and practice all four of the coping steps together.

Procedure

Select the following children to lead the class in the vignette role-play:

Reader: The reader will read the vignette.
Actors: The actors will act out the different roles in the story.
Teacher: You will prompt the actors in the vignette in their roles and any words they might say to each other.
Coach: The coach will instruct the actors in the first two steps of the coping model by prompting them so that they say what they're feeling and then relax and take deep breaths.
Mediator: The mediator will lead the class in brainstorming possible options for the main actor(s) and will help the class determine best choices that are non-violent and are respectful to the self and others.
Director: The director is responsible for leading the actor(s) in acting out the best choice, as determined by the group.

Have the reader proceed to read the vignette to the other children. Have the reader read the vignette again. Prompt the children to act out the roles of the story and any words they might say to each other.

The coach will begin Coping Steps I and II. Have the actors model the first two steps of the coping model by saying I am feeling " ______________ " and then stopping and taking deep breaths and relaxing.

The mediator will begin Coping Step III. Have the whole class describe the main characters' options and best choices, making sure to describe the feelings, options, etc. of all the actors. Record children's descriptions on the chalkboard in four columns: "Feelings," "Options," "Helpful or Harmful," and "Best Choices."

The director will begin Coping Step IV, directing the actor(s) to act out (do) one or more of the best choices as determined by the group (best choices do not harm oneself or other people). If a second actor is utilized, proceed with acting out the best choices for the second actor, with that actor taking the initiative in the role-play. When completed, two or more separate best choices could be acted out.

Vignette—"Give Me Your Lunch Money"

It is Monday morning and you are waiting at the bus stop for the bus. You have your lunch money for the week in your pocket. Two older, tough-looking children come up and start bothering you. Finally one says to you, "Hey punk, give me your lunch money or you're gonna be in big trouble."

STEP IV, EXERCISE 3.
I CAN ACT ON MY BEST CHOICE, Continued
(Ages 8 Through 11)

Introduction

Tell the class that today they will be working on ways to integrate and practice all four of the coping steps together.

Procedure

Select the following children to lead the class in the vignette role-play:

Reader: The reader will read the vignette.
Actors: The actors will act out the different roles in the story.
Teacher: You will prompt the actors in the vignette in their roles and any words they might say to each other.
Coach: The coach will instruct the actors in the first two steps of the coping model by prompting them so that they say what they're feeling and then relax and take deep breaths.
Mediator: The mediator will lead the class in brainstorming possible options for the main actor(s) and will help the class determine best choices that are non-violent and are respectful to the self and others.
Director: The director is responsible for leading the actor(s) in acting out the best choice, as determined by the group.

Have the reader proceed to read the vignette to the other children. Have the reader read the vignette again. Prompt the children to act out the roles of the story and any words they might say to each other.

The coach will begin Coping Steps I and II. Have the actors model the first two steps of the coping model by saying I am feeling " ______________ " and then stopping and taking deep breaths and relaxing.

The mediator will begin Coping Step III. Have the whole class describe the main characters' options and best choices, making sure to describe the feelings, options, etc. of all the actors. Record children's descriptions on the chalkboard in four columns: "Feelings," "Options," "Helpful or Harmful," and "Best Choices."

The director will begin Coping Step IV, directing the actor(s) to act out (do) one or more of the best choices as determined by the group (best choices do not harm oneself or other people). If a second actor is utilized, proceed with acting out the best choices for the second actor, with that actor taking the initiative in the role-play. When completed, two or more separate best choices could be acted out.

Vignette—"Nobody Wants Me"

In P.E. class, the coach has announced you are going to play soccer. He chooses two people to be captains of the teams and tells them to select their team members. When everyone but you has been selected to be on a team, the coach shouts out, "Hey, did you forget about (your name)?" Both team captains roll their eyes and say, "Please don't make us take him/her. We'd like to win for a change."

STEP IV, EXERCISE 4.
I CAN ACT ON MY BEST CHOICE, Continued
(Ages 8 Through 11)

Introduction

Tell the class that today they will be working on ways to integrate and practice all four of the coping steps together.

Procedure

Select the following children to lead the class in the vignette role-play:

Reader: The reader will read the vignette.
Actors: The actors will act out the different roles in the story.
Teacher: You will prompt the actors in the vignette in their roles and any words they might say to each other.
Coach: The coach will instruct the actors in the first two steps of the coping model by prompting them so that they say what they're feeling and then relax and take deep breaths.
Mediator: The mediator will lead the class in brainstorming possible options for the main actor(s) and will help the class determine best choices that are non-violent and are respectful to the self and others.
Director: The director is responsible for leading the actor(s) in acting out the best choice, as determined by the group.

Have the reader proceed to read the vignette to the other children. Have the reader read the vignette again. Prompt the children to act out the roles of the story and any words they might say to each other.

The coach will begin Coping Steps I and II. Have the actors model the first two steps of the coping model by saying I am feeling " ______________ " and then stopping and taking deep breaths and relaxing.

The mediator will begin Coping Step III. Have the whole class describe the main characters' options and best choices, making sure to describe the feelings, options, etc. of all the actors. Record children's descriptions on the chalkboard in four columns: "Feelings," "Options," "Helpful or Harmful," and "Best Choices."

The director will begin Coping Step IV, directing the actor(s) to act out (do) one or more of the best choices as determined by the group (best choices do not harm oneself or other people). If a second actor is utilized, proceed with acting out the best choices for the second actor, with that actor taking the initiative in the role-play. When completed, two or more separate best choices could be acted out.

Vignette—"Making Fun"

You are playing on the parallel bars with two other children at recess time. Both are especially good at gymnastics. When they learn that you can not do a back bend kick over, they begin to laugh and whisper; and you realize they are making fun of you.

STEP IV, EXERCISE 5. I CAN ACT ON MY BEST CHOICE, Continued (Ages 8 Through 11)

Introduction

Tell the class that today they will be working on ways to integrate and practice all four of the coping steps together.

Procedure

Select the following children to lead the class in the vignette role-play:

Reader: The reader will read the vignette.
Actors: The actors will act out the different roles in the story.
Teacher: You will prompt the actors in the vignette in their roles and any words they might say to each other.
Coach: The coach will instruct the actors in the first two steps of the coping model by prompting them so that they say what they're feeling and then relax and take deep breaths.
Mediator: The mediator will lead the class in brainstorming possible options for the main actor(s) and will help the class determine best choices that are non-violent and are respectful to the self and others.
Director: The director is responsible for leading the actor(s) in acting out the best choice, as determined by the group.

Have the reader proceed to read the vignette to the other children. Have the reader read the vignette again. Prompt the children to act out the roles of the story and any words they might say to each other.

The coach will begin Coping Steps I and II. Have the actors model the first two steps of the coping model by saying I am feeling ____________ " and then stopping and taking deep breaths and relaxing.

The mediator will begin Coping Step III. Have the whole class describe the main characters' options and best choices, making sure to describe the feelings, options, etc. of all the actors. Record children's descriptions on the chalkboard in four columns: "Feelings," "Options," "Helpful or Harmful," and "Best Choices."

The director will begin Coping Step IV, directing the actor(s) to act out (do) one or more of the best choices as determined by the group (best choices do not harm oneself or other people). If a second actor is utilized, proceed with acting out the best choices for the second actor, with that actor taking the initiative in the role-play. When completed, two or more separate best choices could be acted out.

Vignette—"You're Late"

Your friend is late. You have been waiting for an hour so both of you can go swimming. Your friend walks up to your front door and knocks. You open the door. Your friend says, "Hi."

Chapter 4

COPING WITH STRESSFUL LIFE SITUATIONS

Pamela Fischer, Ph.D.
Teresa Collins, M.A.

In 1981, David Elkind wrote, "the concept of childhood, so vital to the traditional American way of life, is threatened with extinction . . ." (Elkind, 1981, p. 3). He was referring to the tremendous stress placed on children by a society that pressures them to think, behave, and dress like adults. Fifteen years later, our nation's children are subjected to even more adult life situations than Elkind described. The higher rate of divorce, single-parent families, children living with chronic illness, violence, and poverty have forced children to take on more adult responsibilities and roles. No longer guaranteed protection and safe-keeping by adults, large numbers of children must negotiate their way through difficult life situations alone. Children need coping skills more than ever.

Children, however, receive little instruction in how to cope in healthy ways with these stressful situations. Our society's demand for a quick cure for all of our ills suggests to children that problems can be handled by ingesting a pill or a drink rather than dealing with feelings. Alcohol, tobacco, and tranquilizers have long been modeled as ways to relax and relieve stress. Recently, the prescription antidepressant Prozac has been used increasingly by nondepressed individuals simply to handle everyday pressures and boost confidence levels (Sleek, 1994).

Children living in situations of chronic danger and stress constantly are exposed to unhealthy ways of coping with stress. Drug abuse, violence, and gang membership are common destructive coping strategies used by those living under these conditions. More children are joining gangs for a sense of security. According to Dr. Alan McEvoy, (1994), membership has become a safety tool for youngsters. If you are not a member, you could be a target for violence.

All children need to be taught healthy ways of coping with life's distressing situations. They need skills in both problem-focused coping and emotion-focused coping (Nolen-Hoeksema, 1992). Problem-focused coping skills are most useful when children can exert some control over the situation or make some change (Compas, 1987). Emotion-focused coping skills are used to manage negative feelings in a positive way while one generates a solution to the problem or when the stressor is beyond one's control. If children are given the tools for managing emotions and problem-solving, they will be able to handle stressful situations and negotiate problems competently. In other words, they will develop what Bandura calls self-efficacy (Bandura, 1977), a sense of competency that affects their ability to problem solve, to commit to goals, to perform tasks, and to respond to stress. This sense of competency is an essential factor in emotional well-being and positive mental health. According to Kazdin (1993), "Well-being is not merely the absence of impairment, rather it refers to the presence of personal and interpersonal strengths that promote optimal functioning" (p. 128).

The Emotional Competence Model, described in chapter 2, offers children problem-focused and emotion-focused coping skills to address emotionally distressing situations. Furthermore, it allows children to develop positive skills and social competence that enhance everyday functioning. By following the steps in the model, children can gain a sense of mastery from meeting the demands of the situation while controlling their emotions (Fosson, Martin, & Haley, 1990). The model can be adapted to help children and adolescents cope with a variety of problems and situations. In this chapter are presented some common problems children face and ways in which the model can be practically applied to life situations.

DIVORCE

The Impact of Divorce on Children

In 1990, over one million marriages in the United States ended in divorce, and children were involved in approximately two-thirds of these divorces (Arendell, 1995). Although a leveling off occurred during the 1980s, the divorce rate remains high. If the current trend in divorce continues, three in five first marriages will end in divorce (Martin & Bumpass, 1989).

Divorce is a powerful social stressor that brings significant change for all members of the family, particularly children. Children's long-term adjustments to divorce depend on a variety of individual, family, and environmental factors. Short-term adjustments, however, are more predictable. Parental separation requires children to make immediate changes in their physical living arrangements and adjust to decreased contact with parents, particularly the nonresident parent. Anger, anxiety, sadness, sleep disturbances, distractibility, aggression, and noncompliance commonly are experienced by children at this time (Forehand, Thomas, Wierson, Brody, & Fauber, 1990; Wallerstein & Kelly, 1980).

According to Wallerstein's model (1983a, 1983b), parental divorce requires children to make a series of adjustments: They must acknowledge and accept the situation, deal with loss and feelings of rejection, accept the permanence of the divorce, and give up longings for restoration of the predivorce family. While children are attempting to negotiate these tasks and manage their own feelings of confusion, loss, sadness, and anger, they are likely to encounter a number of other stressors that affect the adjustment process. Reduced parental availability, interparent hostility, limited financial resources, and altered living circumstances are some of the most common situations that confront children of divorcing parents.

Ongoing conflict between former spouses is a major source of stress for children. Divorcing couples, connected by unresolved anger and hurt, purposely or inadvertently may place children in the middle. Children may be used to mediate between parents or be asked to relay information about one parent to another. They also may be subjected to more serious conflicts between parents. Denigration of one parent in front of the children, interference with the other parent's visitations, withholding child support payments, challenging custody arrangements through court proceedings, and child abduction affect children directly and dramatically.

In Arendell's (1995) study of 75 divorced fathers, he found that children frequently were used as pawns in the war between divorcing parents. Half of the custodial fathers reported having used interference with the other parent's visitations as a control strategy. Some control strategies escalate to more serious conflicts displayed in front of children. Confrontations involving violence and threat happened most commonly when children were being transferred between parents. Thus, children were usually witnesses to their parents fighting (Arendell, 1995).

Eighty-five percent of children whose parents are divorced are in the custody of their mother (Arendell, 1995). Thus, children's economic well-being after the divorce is directly related to their mother's economic status. Families headed by a single mother are six times more likely to be impoverished than are families having both parents present (Arendell, 1995). Reduced economic resources often are accompanied by lower quality in housing, neighborhoods, schools, and child care. This change in social status also can mean a loss of social networks and interactions with familiar friends, neighbors, and others. Children may withdraw from peers because of embarrassment about their material losses, and they also may be subjected to increased negative peer pressure that results in performing more socially disapproved acts and violating more school rules (Peterson & Zill, 1986).

Although the literature contains inconsistency concerning the long-term effects of divorce on children, evidence does show that children from divorced families experience poorer adjustment than their peers from intact families (Amato & Keith, 1991). Children of divorced families, especially boys, exhibit higher levels of externalizing behaviors such as aggression and conduct disorders (Camara & Resnick, 1989; Shaw, 1991) and more difficulties in social interactions and academic problems than those from intact families (Guidubaldi, Cleminshaw, Perry, Nastasi, & Lightel, 1986). Parental divorce also has been found to predict unhealthy behaviors such as smoking and drug use in adolescence as well as poor psychological adjustment (Amato & Keith, 1991).

As a result of the significant transitions required of children in a divorcing family, children need both emotion-focused and problem-focused coping strategies to negotiate the demands placed upon them. Children's limited control over many decisions about their new life can make them feel helpless and frustrated (i.e., "It doesn't matter what I do because I have no say so anyway" or "No one cares anyway"). Although children can exert little influence over their post-divorce circumstances, they can learn healthy ways of managing negative emotions. They also can develop an understanding of the divorce and learn to generate solutions to divorce-specific problems. Through role-play and discussion, they can develop an awareness of their feelings and the feelings of others and, perhaps most important, avoid blaming self or others for the divorce.

Gately and Schwebel's Challenge Model (Gately & Schwebel, 1991), designed to describe children's reactions to parental divorce, suggests that children's adjustment during each stage of divorce is shaped by the specific factors of the divorce transition, by their own personal characteristics, and the level of skills and coping resources available to them. Brown, Eichenberger, Portes, and Christensen (1992) suggested that children are more likely to adjust to divorce when they understand the divorce and avoid self-blame. Ankenbrandt (1986) found that children's levels of learned resourcefulness and other cognitive coping skills helped them negotiate divorce adjustment.

Roseby and Deutsch (1985) studied 57 fourth- and fifth-grade students experiencing parental separation or divorce. These students were placed in one of two divorce intervention groups. The experimental group was given training in cognitive social role-taking and assertive communication skills. The control group focused only on feelings about the divorce. The children in the cognitive social role-taking group showed significantly more positive change in their beliefs and attitudes about the divorce than did the control group. Children who received cognitive skills training were less likely to deny their negative feelings or engage in self-blame for the divorce. Evaluation results of other school-based groups developed for children of divorce provide further evidence that teaching children anger control, relaxation techniques, and cognitive-behavioral skills for problem solving can reduce the negative effects of the postdivorce adjustment period (Pedro-Carroll & Cowen, 1985; Stolberg & Garrison, 1985; Stolberg & Mahler, 1994).

Strategies for Helping Children Cope with Parental Divorce

The use of the Emotional Competence Model teaches children to recognize and cope with the unpleasant feelings and situations that accompany parental divorce. Presented below is an example of how the model can be adapted to help children deal with some of the common feelings experienced in this situation.

Step I—Accept. Situations that accompany a divorce generate a variety of feelings often difficult for children to accept. Acceptance of feelings, however, is the foundation for coping with them.

Confusion

Situation: *"One day I want to live with Mom, and one day I want to live with Dad. . . ."*
Acceptance: *"I feel confused about where I want to live and who I want to live with."*

Hurt

Situation: *"Sometimes I have to listen to my mother make hateful comments about my father."*
Acceptance: *"I feel hurt when my mother calls my father names or says that he is worthless."*

Lonely

Situation: *"Since I live with my mother most of the time, sometimes I feel really lonely without my Dad."*
Acceptance: *"I miss my Dad when I am not with him."*

Angry

Situation: *"Because my parents have to pay for two places to live, I don't have money for some things I used to. It's just not fair for me to have to give up things just because they can't get along."*
Acceptance: *"I feel angry when I don't get to have as many things as I did before."*

Step II—Pause. Pausing to gain composure after acknowledging an unpleasant emotional state is a key to coping effectively. Comments and messages children can give to themselves are listed below:

I need to pause and take time out.
I need to relax for a moment.
I need to get control of myself.
I need to pause so I can decide what to do with this feeling.
I need to relax and take a deep breath.
I need to breathe deeply and count to 10.

Step III—Think. Children can use problem-solving strategies for dealing with difficult emotions and life situations following a divorce. This process of problem solving includes generating options to help themselves without hurting others. The process of generating those options and evaluating them is illustrated in the following example.

What is the situation?	*What am I feeling?*	*I need to pause and relax.*	*What could I do in this situation?*	*Will this action help me or harm me?*
My mother walks in my room and tells me that it is time to pack my bag because my father is coming to get me in an hour. I am busy playing a game with my friend.	Sad Angry Hurt Frustrated	I decide to take some deep breaths.	Yell at my mother.	Harm
			Call my father and tell him I don't want to go.	Harm
			Tell my mother what I'm feeling.	Help
			Pack my bag.	Help
			Save game to play later.	Help
			Bargain with my mother or call my father for more time.	Difficult to know.

Step IV—Do. Acting on the best choice means choosing to *do* something now that I believe could help me without hurting me or others. Sometimes a choice must be acted upon before I know whether it can really help.

In the previous example, some possible best choices might include the following:

1. Bargain with my mother or father for more time to play the game.
2. Pack my bag.
3. Save the game to play later.

LOSS THROUGH DEATH OR ILLNESS

The Impact of Traumatic Loss on Children

Grief is a complex set of emotions that includes sadness, despair, and anger. Typically we think of grief occurring as a result of losing a loved one through death; however, grief can occur when one experiences "any major change in a familiar pattern of behavior" (James & Cherry, 1988, p. 4). Serious illness or death of a parent or any event that brings a significant change in lifestyle can trigger a grief reaction.

While all of us find loss a painful experience, children may have a particularly difficult time coping with death and loss for a number of reasons. Children are not experienced in expressing their feelings and may be around individuals who are ill-prepared to help them deal with loss. They may be told to "Buck up," "Get over it," or "Big boys/girls don't cry." Their feelings may be directly challenged by hearing adults say, "Don't be sad. You should be grateful that you had him/her for so long."

"The natural dependency of childhood along with the potential for animistic and magical thinking make children particularly vulnerable to prolonged adverse psychological sequelae following an important loss" (Koocher & Gudas, 1992, p. 1029). Myths and certain religious beliefs about death are often confusing to children. Children may hear that "Grandpa is now an angel," "He's gone to sleep," or "He's gone to a better place." The common use of metaphors when talking about the deceased can be anxiety-producing, frightening, and baffling to children. When children inquire about a death and are told, for instance, that "Grandpa's gone," or "We've lost Grandpa," they likely expect him to show up later.

Likewise, many adults believe that it is better for the child not to know about the course and ramifications of a parent's illness (Titler, Cohen, & Craft, 1991). These adults tend to shield children from information about an ill parent (Nicholson, Titler, Montgomery, Kleiber, Craft, Halm, & Buckwalter, 1993). As a result, children are left to form their own conclusions about what is happening to their parent; and they often end up feeling anxious, frightened, angry, and confused. When a parent dies and the child has not been informed of the seriousness of the illness, there can be a sense of betrayal.

Additionally, parental illness or death may result in the child assuming adult-like roles. Johnston, Martin, Martin and Gumaer (1992) found that in the case of parental illness, role reversals may occur as the sick parent becomes more child-like, and the child begins to assume a parental role. Adult-like behaviors often are reinforced by parents, relatives, and hospital staff who believe that the child is able to understand fully their parent's illness. This assumption is likely to compromise the developmental tasks of the child. Children may express their confusion and frustration with all of these life changes by acting out or by using drugs or alcohol (Drotar, 1994; Gallo, Breitmayer, Knafl, & Zoeller, 1992; Glass, 1985).

Strategies for Helping Children Cope with Death or Illness

Children need assistance in learning ways to cope with loss and death. They also need help in maintaining a sense of normalcy in their daily routines. As with other stressors facing children, children will be helped by accepting and coping with their feelings in a healthy manner. The four steps of the Emotional Competence Model give them a strategy for doing so.

Step I—Accept.

Frightened

Situation: *"I saw my mother being wheeled into the operating room, and I wanted to run away and hide."*
Acceptance: *"I felt scared when I saw my mother go into the operating room."*

Anger

Situation: *"At the father-son baseball game, my dad had to sit on the sidelines and watch."*
Acceptance: *"I felt angry that my dad couldn't play in the game like the other dads.*

Embarrassed

Situation: *"Everybody stares at us when we walk in a restaurant or go to the mall."*
Acceptance: *"I feel embarrassed when people stare at us because my mom's hair has fallen out since she started taking chemotherapy."*

Sad

Situation: *"I sometimes cry when I see other girls out with their moms going shopping and having fun."*
Acceptance: *"I feel sad because I don't have my mom to do things with anymore."*

Step II—Pause. Pausing to gain composure after acknowledging an unpleasant emotional state is a key to coping effectively. Comments and messages children can give to themselves include the following:

I need to pause and take time out.
I need to relax for a moment.
I need to get control of myself.
I need to pause so I can decide what to do with this feeling.
I need to relax and take a deep breath.
I need to breathe deeply and count to 10.

Step III—Think. Children can use problem-solving strategies for dealing with difficult emotions and life situations following loss through death and illness. This process of problem solving includes generating options to help themselves without hurting others. The process of generating those options and evaluating them is illustrated in the example shown here.

What is the situation?	*What am I feeling?*	*I need to pause and relax.*	*What could I do in this situation?*	*Will this action help me or harm me?*
My dad had a heart attack and died suddenly. If something happens to Mom, "I won't have anybody!"	Frightened Worried	I decide to take some deep breaths.	Keep my feelings to myself so I won't bother Mom. She's worried enough already.	Harm
			"Be a man" and handle it. Only wimps are afraid.	Harm
			Talk to my Mom about my concerns.	Help
			Make a list of adults in my life who care for me.	Help
			Make a scrapbook of special memories of me and Dad so I won't feel so lonely.	Help

Step IV—Do. Acting on the best choice means choosing to *do* something now that I believe could help me without hurting me or others. Sometimes a choice must be acted upon before I know whether it can really help.

In the previous example, some possible best choices might include the following:

1. Talk with Mom about the situation and explain my concerns to her.
2. Make a list of all the adults who love me and care for me to help me remember that I'm not alone.
3. Make a scrapbook of special memories about Dad so I won't feel so lonely.

CHILD ILLNESS

The Impact of Chronic Illness on Children

Chronic physical illness is also a major life stressor for increasing numbers of children. Advances in medical treatment have led to children with life-threatening conditions living longer. Children with serious illnesses experience difficulties in coping with pain, physical limitations, treatment regimens, depression, anxiety, and school. Hospitalization also provides many stressors. Children may be unfamiliar with the hospital environment and its personnel. They may resist parting from their parent prior to surgery. Children also may react negatively to disruption of typical routines, loss of control over daily events, greater dependency on others, and misconceptions about the purpose of their hospitalization (Peterson, 1989; Siegel & Hudson, 1992).

In the past, children often were not told about their upcoming medical procedures. There was a belief that children were not mature enough cognitively to understand and remember information regarding their illness (Burbach & Peterson, 1986; Eiser & Eiser, 1987). This belief contradicts that of most professionals who concede that sensitive and developmentally appropriate preparation is beneficial to children (Eiser & Eiser, 1987; Schultheis, Peterson, & Selby, 1987). Children are likely to describe feeling sad, angry, confused, scared, or a combination of these feelings when confronted with illness.

Children's thoughts and feelings about their illness and its treatment vary. The condition of their health, upcoming procedures, or changes at home or school all factor into their total experience. Children who are experiencing a high level of distress are likely to be noncompliant with treatments. Research, however, suggests that children can reduce their stress level by being given an opportunity to learn about their illness and discuss their thoughts and feelings.

Illness may be the result of a malfunction of a body part, but health also can be compromised by psychological distress. Eiser and Eiser (1987) believed that health care providers need to "foster empathy, facilitate explanations of illness and medical procedures, and improve health education" (p. 283) in order to relieve stress in children. The literature consistently supports the finding that younger children particularly, who probably understand less about their illness or the procedures, tend to be at risk for developing emotional and behavioral problems both during and following hospitalization (Siegel & Hudson, 1992). Interventions should focus on enabling the child to deal with specific stressful situations and the development of appropriate coping skills.

Strategies for Helping Children Cope with Illness

Relaxation, self-instruction, and imagery distraction are effective in decreasing a child's anxiety while enhancing compliance with treatment (Peterson & Shigetomi, 1981). The Emotional Competence Model for coping can support children undergoing a wide range of medical procedures. Those include relatively painless procedures such as physical examinations, but they also can include major interventions such as open-heart surgeries. Instruction in specific coping activities gives patients a technique to minimize the impact of aversive stimuli. This technique also can modify one's assessment of the event and thereby alter the emotional reaction (Schultheis et al., 1987).

Aside from the specific medical procedures, the Emotional Competence Model also can be utilized to assist children in coping with a wide variety of feelings and situations that children with chronic illnesses are likely to face. Some examples of utilizing the model are listed below.

Step I—Accept.

Angry

Situation: *"All my friends are doing something fun over Christmas break but I have to go to the hospital."*
Acceptance: *"I am angry that I have to spend my Christmas break in the hospital."*

Frightened

Situation: *"I've seen an operating room on television. It has huge lights and lots of weird-looking machines that they hook you up to. Many people die in the operating room."*
Acceptance: *"When I think about being in the operating room, I become very frightened."*

Sad

Situation: *"I wish I could have a 'normal' life like other kids."*
Acceptance: *"I am sad that my illness prevents me from having a life like the other kids."*

Frustrated

Situation: *"It seems that every time I start feeling pretty good, something goes wrong and I end up back in the hospital."*
Acceptance: *"I am frustrated that my illness interferes with my life."*

Step II—Pause. Pausing to gain composure after acknowledging an unpleasant emotional state is a key to coping effectively. Comments and messages children can give to themselves include the following:

I need to pause and take time out.
I need to relax for a moment.
I need to get control of myself.
I need to pause so I can decide what to do with this feeling.
I need to relax and take a deep breath.
I need to breathe deeply and count to 10.

Step III—Think. A practical example of how Emotional Competence coping techniques can be used to help a child undergoing a medical procedure is shown here.

What is the situation?	*What am I feeling?*	*I need to pause and relax.*	*What could I do in this situation?*	*Will this action help or harm me?*
David, a reluctant 5-year-old boy, walks to the lab, eases into the chair, and hesitantly offers the nurse his arm.	Anxious Scared The nurse acknowledges and accepts his feelings as a natural part of his reaction to the procedure. By the nurse's acceptance of David's feelings, she helps him accept them as well.	The nurse instructs David to take deep breaths as if he were a balloon letting all of the air come out.	David constructs the image of a plane flying, dipping in and out of the clouds. As he dreams of flying, he looks away from the needle and relaxes his arm while the nurse draws his blood.	Help

Step IV—Do. Acting on the best choice means choosing to *do* something now that I believe could help me without hurting me or others. Sometimes a choice must be acted upon before I know whether it can really help.

In the previous example, best choices for relaxation and distraction during the medical procedure might include the following:

1. Take deep breaths in and out as if I were a balloon.
2. Construct the image of a flying plane, dipping in and out of the clouds.

ABUSE AND NEGLECT

The Impact of Abuse and Neglect on Children

Children suffer more victimization than do adults. This victimization includes experiences of more conventional crimes and more family violence. There are also some crimes that are unique to children, such as family abduction (Finkelhor & Dziuba-Leatherman, 1994). Children are more prone to victimization than adults because of their weak, small physical stature and dependent nature (Finkelhor & Dziuba-Leatherman, 1994). They also are not able to make certain choices for themselves regarding whom they associate with, where they live, or where they go to school. Many of these choices are made for them by adult family members. It is not surprising, then, that more victimizations of children occur at the hands of relatives (Finkelhor & Dziuba-Leatherman, 1994). Parents are the primary perpetrators of neglect and psychological maltreatment (Sedlak, 1991). They also represent 51% of those who commit sexual abuse of children. Abuse that stems from parental maltreatment is likely to cause long-term developmental impairments that persist into adulthood (Kempe & Kempe, 1978).

The type and severity of abuse are related to the child's level of development and age at the time of the abuse and/or neglect. For example, small children are more vulnerable to death and serious harm as a result of inflicted blows while older children suffer more penetrative abuse (Kerns & Rutter, 1991). Regardless of age, maltreatment during childhood is likely to have serious short- and long-term effects on children's mental health functioning. Child victims are likely to have low trust of others, poor moral development, and aggressive behaviors (Wolfe, 1987). Sexually abused children have a greater risk for substance abuse and psychiatric disorders (Scott, 1992). Adult victims of child abuse and neglect are likely to report having a limited ability to relate to others, poor self-esteem, fear of failure, difficulties in cognitive learning, and an inability to cope with ordinary problems in daily living (Hackett, 1993).

Childhood victimization also increases the risk of becoming a perpetrator of crime, violence, and abuse. Many studies have found that abused children direct aggression toward their peers and family members (Wolfe, 1987). At the same time, children who are abused and/or neglected are also more likely to be seen as avoidant and resistant (Crouch & Milner, 1993). They often choose to remain isolated from their peers due to feeling betrayed, powerless, and stigmatized (Browne & Finkelhor, 1986). They are likely to report feeling sad, scared, angry, and confused by their parent's actions.

Strategies for Helping Children Cope with Abuse and Neglect

Children dealing with abuse or neglect need to legitimize their feelings and gain a sense of competency and control. Learning to accept their feelings, relax, and explore new ways to help themselves could prepare children for what lies ahead when they begin to disclose the specifics regarding their maltreatment. Although it cannot realistically help children generate solutions to solve the problem of victimization, it can help them generate ideas about where they can get help. In situations where verbal or physical abuse does not reach criminal stature, children also may use this coping strategy to reduce or minimize the amount of abuse they receive.

Step I—Accept. Situations that accompany abuse often generate feelings that children have difficulty accepting. Acceptance of feelings, however, is the foundation for coping with them. Examples of common emotional states that abused and/or neglected children experience and examples of acceptance of those feelings are listed below.

Frightened

Situation: *"Every time I see my uncle walk in the door, I get sick to my stomach."*
Acceptance: *"I am scared of what my uncle may do to me."*

Helpless

Situation: *"When my mother starts to call me names, I want to tell her to stop, but I know it won't do any good."*
Acceptance: *"I feel helpless about getting my mother to stop calling me names."*

Confused

Situation: *"If my dad says that he loves me, then why does he hit me?"*
Acceptance: *"I feel confused about my Dad's behavior towards me."*

Angry

Situation: *"I can never ask a friend to come to my house because I never know what will be going on—who will be in a bad mood."*
Acceptance: *"I feel angry that my home life is so unpredictable."*

Step II—Pause. Pausing to gain composure after acknowledging an unpleasant emotional state is a key to coping effectively. Comments and messages children can give to themselves are listed below.

I need to pause and take time out.
I need to relax for a moment.
I need to get control of myself.
I need to pause so I can decide what to do with this feeling.
I need to relax and take a deep breath.
I need to breathe deeply and count to 10.

Step III—Think. Children can use problem-solving strategies for dealing with difficult emotions and life situations involving abuse and neglect. This process of problem solving includes generating options to help themselves without hurting others. The process of generating those options and evaluating them is illustrated in the following example.

What is the situation?	*What am I feeling?*	*I need to pause and relax.*	*What could I do in this situation?*	*Will this action help me or harm me?*
My dad starts slapping me when he's had a bad day at work.	Angry Confused	I decide to take a deep breath to get control of myself.	Talk to my dad about his mood.	Harm
			Talk with my mom.	Don't know.
			Go to my room and stay out of his way when he's in an angry mood.	May help.
			Go on a bike ride until Dad cools down from his bad day at work.	May help.

Step IV—Do. Acting on the best choice means choosing to *do* something now that I believe could help me without hurting me or others. Sometimes a choice must be acted upon before we know whether it can really help.

In the example above, some possible best choices might include the following:

1. Talking with Mom.
2. Going to my room and staying out of Dad's way.
3. Going on a bike ride.

LIVING IN A VIOLENT WORLD

The Impact of Violence and Trauma on Children

Children are growing up in America with firsthand knowledge of violence and disaster. The United States has the highest per capita incidence of interpersonal violence of any nation not actively engaged in civil war (Lykken, 1993). Violence in many American cities has provided scenes that look similar to the war zones of Beirut, Belfast, and Mozambique (Garbarino, Dubrow, Kostelny, & Pardo, 1992). As the incidences of domestic violence in the United States increase, children are becoming increasingly familiar with stabbings, shootings, wife battering, and acts of random violence. What they do not experience personally, the media bring to them in detail. Exposure to drugs, gangs, guns, ethnic prejudice, terrorist activities, and natural disasters creates both a fear of and an adaptation to the horrors of violence.

As children repeatedly witness violence first hand and through the media, their view of the world as safe and predictable is shattered. As a result, children may experience fear, anxiety, anger, nightmares, difficulty with concentration, or social withdrawal. Some may act younger than their age or complain of physical symptoms such as headaches, stomachaches, or eating problems.

Living with violence also invites immunity to violent acts. Children forced to cope with chronic danger may adapt in ways that are dysfunctional. They may cope with danger by adopting a world view that may be dysfunctional in normal situations (Garbarino, Kostelny, & Dubrow, 1991). Research has found that children who are exposed to violent events become more aggressive with their peers (Attar, Guerra, & Tolan, 1994). Repeated observations of violence also may impact the child's internal standards of appropriate behavior. The child may begin to normalize and condone the presence of violent acts that may lead to a lifetime impact. For example, violent preschool- and school-age children are prone to violence in adolescence and adulthood (Wall & Holden, 1994).

Evidence indicates that children can be taught to inhibit their aggression when the setting requires the control of aggression (Lore & Schultz, 1993). In fact, interventions to control aggression are most successful when they are used with young children. These interventions include interpersonal problem-solving training, cognitive strategies, and social skills training (Prinz, Blechman, & Dumas, 1994).

Slaby (1994) said that violence can be prevented most easily by using intervention programs designed to strengthen the habits of thinking with youngsters in the early stages of life. In a recent study by the Education Development Center in California, thinking patterns of 17-year-old inmates convicted of rape and attempted murder or assault were compared to 17-year-old high school students. "What we found is they [inmates] do not think thoroughly at all about violence and they don't have the skill to think of alternatives. When put in conflict situations the inmates didn't think consequentially or pose alternative solutions" (Slaby, 1994, p. 37). Thus teaching children problem-solving skills is essential in reducing violent and aggressive acts.

Emotion-focused coping skills also can be helpful when children need to address their fears and anxieties about living in a violent and traumatic world. School-age children often become intensely preoccupied with the details of a traumatic event and can benefit from talking about what happened in the context of their normal routines. Talking allows assimilation of the traumatic event into the child's understanding of his or her situation. While discussing the event with the child, parents, teachers, counselors, and other adults can set an example by the way they respond to the crisis.

Strategies for Helping Children Cope with Violent and Traumatic Events

Ironically, as this chapter was being written, the Alfred P. Murrah Federal Building in Oklahoma City was bombed, killing 168 people. For the first time, many of our community's children were exposed to a senseless act of extreme violence. Children expressed a variety of emotions and behaviors about this event. Many exhibited anxiety, irritability, fear, and increased dependency. Many teachers reported behavior difficulties and a general restlessness among students.

The Emotional Competence Model proved to be a helpful strategy in assisting children to cope with this disaster. Children were encouraged to express and talk about their feelings. Many children came up with ideas about what they could do to help themselves and others feel better. Many pictures and letters were sent to rescue workers, family members, and hospitals. Many children's groups planted a tree or garden in memory of the victims. Bake sales and fund raisers were held to raise money to donate to the family members of the victims. An outpouring of concern, support, and assistance came from our own community, state, and country. Children watched, participated, and experienced how doing something to help themselves also can help others.

Figures 4.1 and 4.2 are an interview guide and sample of a record sheet that were used to help children cope with their feelings about this disaster. This guide can be used to assist children anywhere who are trying to cope with their feelings following a disaster.

LISTEN TO THE CHILDREN INTERVIEW GUIDE (For Use Following a Disaster or Community Trauma)

Purpose

Listen to the Children Interview Guide is an interview with school-age children to determine their current status and condition. The theme is to listen carefully and record their answers.

Preparation

It can be helpful if two people conduct the interview. In that way, one person can record the children's answers on the blackboard, while the other can record them on the record sheet. The two individuals can be a teacher and DARE officer, a teacher and a parent, or others.

Instructions

1. Introduce yourself and tell where you are from. If you have worked in the schools this year, tell the children what you did. Tell them that your job today is to help people by talking with them and listening to them.
2. Tell the children that you want to learn from them about their thoughts and feelings since the disaster occurred.
3. Tell the children that you want to learn from them, and ask them if they will help you. (Try to get as many nods as possible.)
4. For each of the following two questions, record and write answers on the chalkboard (e.g., one person can record answers on the record sheet [Figure 4.2], and one person can write answers on the chalkboard):

> "Tell me (us) what you understand about the ______________ (i.e., specific disaster). How did it happen and why?"

> "Now, can you tell me (us) what kinds of feelings you have had? I would like to know about the easy feelings, such as feeling happy, proud, or safe if you had them, and any hard feelings such as scared or sad or angry." List the hard and easy feelings on the chalkboard.

5. After listing the hard feelings on the board, have the class brainstorm about the things that they could do or already have done (i.e., choices) to help themselves feel better. Write the word *choices* on the chalkboard and record their answers. If some of the choices do not seem healthy (i.e., they harm the self or others), take

Figure 4.1. Listen to the Children Interview Guide (for Use Following a Disaster or Community Trauma).

the next step and write the words *best choices* on the chalkboard. Explain to the class that best choices help and do not harm the children themselves or others. Tell the children that not everyone will have the same best choice. Then record best choices from the class.

6. Finally, ask the children what others could do to help them most. Record their suggestions for parents and school staff to utilize (#4 on sample Record Sheet, Figure 4.2).

7. Thank the children and prepare to leave. Tell them that you will give information to the school staff, the parents, and the children themselves after you and the children have completed these "listening sessions."

Figure 4.1. Continued.

Grade: ______________________ School: ______________________

LISTEN TO THE CHILDREN RECORD SHEET

1. UNDERSTANDING OF THE DISASTER

How did it happen?

Why did it happen?

2. THOUGHTS AND FEELINGS

Thoughts:

Easy Feelings: Hard Feelings:

3. CHOICES AND BEST CHOICES

Choices: Best Choices:

4. WHAT OTHERS CAN DO TO HELP

Suggestions for Parents: Suggestions for Teachers and School Staff:

5. ADDITIONAL INTERVIEW NOTES

Figure 4.2. Sample of the Listen to the Children Record Sheet.

SECTION II
BUILDING MUSCLES FOR MENTAL HEALTH

Chapter 5

THE INGREDIENTS OF STRONG MENTAL MUSCLES

We usually think of muscles as parts of our body that contribute to our forcefulness, our stamina, and our vigor. Muscles provide the strength and power for motion. They develop gradually as we mature, and they need to be exercised consistently to reach their optimal potential.

Analogous to these physical muscles are "mental muscles." We cannot see them, but we believe they serve a function similar to physical muscles. They provide the strength for emotional health by serving as the raw materials for helping us move and relate effectively in the world around us. Similar to their counterpart in the physical realm, they develop slowly and only with much practice and exercise.

Exercising and strengthening mental muscles is much like building a resource bank that can be drawn upon and used when demands are placed upon us. The more resources we have in the bank and the more we exercise them, the less likely we are to become bankrupt in times of stress. We can build our resource bank of healthy mental muscles by learning ways of thinking and living that help us care for ourselves and establish more caring relationships with others.

The roots of this ability to care for ourselves and others grow out of learning how to sustain a healthy connection to our own selves and out of learning how to differentiate ourselves from others (Bellingham, Cohen, Jones, & Spanoil, 1989). Concretely, this means learning ways to know and understand our own thoughts, feelings, and values. It also means learning how to separate our thoughts, feelings, and values from those of others. This knowledge of ourselves provides us with the substance of our identity or who we are as persons. As we acknowledge and respect what we think, feel, and value, we assert, validate, and differentiate our individual lives and develop the resources for effective relationships (Dlugokinski, 1990).

The process of differentiating ourselves from others is often described as psychological separation or individuation. As we psychologically separate, we develop personal boundaries that provide space between *me* and *not me*. Initially, we begin this separation process as we develop independent thought and action from our own parents, but we continue to separate our identity from that of others throughout our lifetime.

Developmental theorists have emphasized the importance of the development of a personal self for healthy adjustment and emotional well-being. Psychoanalytic theory (Blos, 1979; Mahler, 1968), Heinz Kohut's developmental self theory (Kohut, 1971), Erikson's psychosocial theory (Erikson, 1968), and family systems theory (Olson, Russell, & Sprenkle, 1983) all emphasize the importance of the emerging young person taking more responsibility for emotional, behavioral, and cognitive coping while becoming progressively more independent from his/her parents. According to these theorists, this process takes place through a series of developmental tasks that, if mastered, help to free the child from an enmeshed and dependent existence, and toward a healthy, adjusted, and unique personal identity.

Healthy adjustment includes similar tasks for all of us. The culmination of these tasks is the development of a differentiated, competent, unique individual. The self that is differentiated also needs to be valued and respected; however, valuing the self does not mean practicing selfishness. Individuals need not only to value and respect themselves but also to develop healthy and compassionate ways of relating to others.

Although the two needs for individuation and social responsibility are often seen as competing priorities, it might be more realistic to conceive of both as essential and complimentary ingredients to healthy human functioning (Ryan & Lynch, 1989). In this scheme then, self-development and the development of personal boundaries are intimately related to promoting healthy connectedness to others. As the self becomes better defined and articulated, the individual becomes more capable of connecting with others without intrusiveness or isolation.

Thus, the evolution of a unique, valued self is congruent with healthy and compassionate relationships with others. These two developmental processes evolve in an interactive, reciprocally balanced, mutually facilitating fashion from birth through senescence (Blatt & Schichman, 1983). An inadequately developed personal boundary system often sacrifices both personal emotional well-being and effective relationships with others. If one sacrifices self-development, interpersonal relationships also suffer (Guisinger & Blatt, 1994).

This parallel development of a healthy self and healthy relationships with others makes sense when we look at the area of personal and social responsibility. Responsibilities are most likely to be carried out and adhered to when they are clearly articulated and well-defined. For example, when a group of individuals sees a person who is pleading for help or assistance, often no one in the group stops to help this individual because the sense of responsibility remains ill-defined and fuzzy. When any one of these individuals alone, however, encounters the person in need, he/she is more likely to stop and assist because the sense of personal responsibility is clear.

The same process occurs in emotional development. As the self becomes more well-differentiated emotionally, there is a clearer view of *me* and *not me*. This, in turn, also leads to a clearer articulation of responsibility for the self and caretaking activities for others. When the emotional self is clearly defined, resourceful, and expressive, social responsibilities to others are more likely to be met. Those responsibilities to others are met because they become more clearly defined and the individual has greater resources in the self to assist others. When both individuals have clearly delineated personal and social responsibilities, the healthiest relationships can occur.

This psychological process has various practical implications for parents, family systems, and educational environments that serve children. We need to teach children ways to know and express themselves as well as ways to respect others. We need to delineate clearly both personal and social responsibilities. For example, we need to teach children to be responsible for knowing and expressing their own emotions, *and* we need to teach them to be respectful of but not responsible for the emotions of others. When others are in emotional pain, we need to find ways for children to be compassionate and supportive; however, we do not need to teach children to cope *for* those individuals or to try to manage someone else's feelings.

We also need to teach children to differentiate between their personal space and the space of others. Children have a personal responsibility to maintain their own space. This includes their room, their body, their desk at school, and others areas of personal surroundings and possessions. They have a right to become angry if their space is violated, and they need to know that others have a right to their anger when their space is violated. They have a social responsibility to respect the personal space of others. Social responsibility, then, goes hand in hand with accepting and experiencing personal responsibility.

Building strong muscles for mental and emotional health involves learning and exercising ways of thinking and living that lead to a well-differentiated self respectful of others. The elements that contribute to this muscle-building process for elementary school children might be conceived of as learning and exercising skills to

develop the self,
respect the self and others,
build strength through habits, and
balance work and play.

DEVELOPING THE SELF

Erik Erikson (1968) proposed and developed a well-differentiated theory of personality development that involved eight stages of differentiation of the self. In each stage the self grows stronger and more capable of expressing itself in an authoritative and productive manner. During the first stage, the infant needs to feel a sense of safety for the "I" to exist. Once this sense of trust is established, the toddler can begin to develop a separate sense of autonomy and can begin primitive differentiation from parents. In the preschool years, this developing sense of "I" begins to explore the world in an assertive fashion. If this assertiveness is not squelched, the child develops a sense of initiative and believes that the "I" can take active steps to relate to the world. In the elementary school years, the "I" begins to develop a sense of industry and often compares him/herself with other children. School-age children compete in talents, work products, and physical ability. At times they also can be cruelly competitive by engaging in name calling and other methods of pointing out each other's weaknesses. If the child survives this entry into the peer world and believes that he/she can fit in to the larger society, a sense of industry, competence, and belonging is developed.

Erikson describes each of these four stages of self-development as involving a crisis, or a turning point, for the individual. If the turning point is managed successfully, the child develops a more differentiated and competent sense of self. The stages build upon one another in a stepwise fashion. The "I" that learns that it is safe to exist, can go on to learn about existing autonomously, then to initiate activity, and then to feel a sense of competence in its own actions. The risk at each stage is that the "I" will not advance and will experience basic mistrust instead of safety, shame instead of autonomy, guilt instead of initiative, and inferiority instead of competence. Erikson stipulates that an individual needs a basic or minimal amount of these positive self-attributes for development to proceed effectively.

In his view of the developing person, Erikson primarily concentrates on the emotional growth of the evolving self. The emotional self, in Erikson's system, is represented as a series of building blocks that can only be as strong and stable as the lowest blocks in the structure. With each stage of basically positive development, the "I" puts a block in the structure and comes closer to a competent and capable personal self. Although it is optimal to think of the "I" as developing towards healthy emotional maturity, it does not always happen. Development of the emotional "I" can get stuck along the way.

At the same time that emotional growth is occurring, the thoughts of the self are also slowly differentiating and becoming more sophisticated. Piaget (1963) traced how the child's thought process evolves. Gradually the infant moves from sensory and motor ways of understanding the world to the evolution of logical and abstract thinking in adolescence. In Piaget's framework, the self, or "I," becomes increasingly capable and competent in relating to the world effectively as the development of thinking proceeds. Each stage of development adds a new dimension of cognitive skills to the child's ability to comprehend the world. Piaget points out that there is an orderly, predictable progression of abilities in cognition; however, for the thinking "I" to achieve optimal cognitive development, both adult direction and active experiencing or practice are essential.

Piaget's emphasis on active experience is worthy of special mention. In his theoretical framework, the "thinking" self learns the meaning of objects and activities in life by acting on them. For example, the young child learns the meaning of a rubber ball by touching it, holding it, bouncing it, and actively engaging and experiencing that ball. Only by acting on that ball does the child learn to understand the meaning of a rubber ball. The structure of the mind progresses, then, through active experience with objects in the world. Active participation and exploration by the learner is essential to the learning process because the child's thought process does not mature through a passive accumulation of information.

Piaget's conceptualization may be helpful, then, in understanding why information strategies alone are ineffective in prevention of dysfunctional behavior (Schaps et al., 1988). We cannot pour knowledge and action strategies into the mind of a child. We must actively engage the child's thought process for true learning to occur.

Kohlberg (1984) focused more on the evolution of moral understanding and value acquisition. Infants and preschool children are almost amoral in their thinking. Later, values and "rights and wrongs" are defined for the elementary school child by significant adults at home and at school. Some individuals never get beyond following the rules of others. In the highest evolution of a moral self, however, an individual can attain the ability to differentiate right from wrong based on absolute principles rather than simply parroting the rules of others.

Children learn what to value by how they live and by observing how adults live. They learn the value of a moral principle by living that way themselves. For example, children learn the value of cooperation by observing and practicing cooperation. Thus, the highest evolution of the moral "I" can only be attained if there are appropriate role models and opportunities to practice and live those principles.

In summary, to develop as whole and self-reliant individuals, children need to understand their own thoughts, feelings, and values and to develop their skills gradually in each of these areas (Glenn & Nelson, 1988). Jack Pransky (1991) viewed this type of self-understanding and development as a critical component of a "healthy self-perception," a key factor in the prevention of a variety of personal and interpersonal dysfunctions. In essence, a person with a healthy self-perception is respectful of his/her unique identity, is competent, and experiences control over his/her own life.

RESPECTING THE SELF AND OTHERS

Closely related to developing the self is acquiring an ability to value the self and others. Although we have differentiated these ideas for purposes of programming content, they are intertwined in developmental theory (Erikson, 1968; Glenn & Nelson, 1988; Mahler, 1968). The marriage of these two concepts also is illustrated by Jack Pransky's (1991) ideas of a "healthy self-perception" and Eric Dlugokinski's (1990) model for "caring connections." Both authors emphasize the interconnectedness between developing the self, valuing the self, and valuing others. Caring connections espouses a respectful connection with our own thoughts, feelings, and values while simultaneously listening to and respecting the thoughts, feelings, and values of others. In essence, this includes an ability to care for ourselves (esteem ourselves) and care about others (esteem others). We learn how to esteem ourselves and others by seeing others practice it, by living in an atmosphere that fosters it, and by practicing this esteeming process ourselves.

The highly accredited work of the California Task Force on Self-Esteem (1990) highlighted the importance of self-esteem to social and emotional development. This task force met for three years with 29 members and reviewed thousands of scientific documents and testimonies. The findings of this panel have fueled the growth of a national self-esteem movement that has encouraged 20 other states to plan ways to cultivate self-esteem in their own area. The findings are simple: Self-esteem acts like a social vaccine. As long as you have it in your system, you can ward off a host of society's ills. The California Task Force (1990) incorporated the notion that self-esteem also includes esteem for others. They define self-esteem as "appreciating our own worth and importance, and having the character to be accountable for ourselves and act responsibly towards others" (p. 1).

Coopersmith (1967) defined self-esteem as the thought and feeling of being good enough. This experience of being good enough is a subjective experience and relates to the individual's ability to believe that he/she is worthy of a satisfying life. To experience a sense of worthiness, or feeling of being good enough, one must believe that he/she is valuable as a human being. This belief in one's own value comes from inner contentment rather than from such externals as peer praises and flashy possessions (Urbanska, 1991).

When we are infants and young children, self-esteem is mostly given to us by others through the way they value us. During our childhood years, however, adults also can empower us by teaching us ways to value ourselves. Adults can guide us to teach ourselves to reward hard work with relaxation and to value ourselves enough not to submit ourselves to dangerous drugs or high-risk endeavors. As we grow and develop, we can learn to practice more of these habits that value us. We can choose consciously to be compassionate to ourselves and to others.

To build strong mental muscles for our children, then, we need to develop exercises and daily rituals that assist children in empowering their own lives through valuing themselves. Living in self-esteem is a habit that feels more comfortable the more we practice it.

BUILDING STRENGTH THROUGH HABITS

It is easy to underestimate the power of a habit. Habits become a part of our identity, who we are, and how we define ourselves. Some habits are beneficial to us. We have a usual way, for example, of combing our hair, brushing our teeth, opening doors, adjusting our glasses, or opening mail. Habitual ways of accomplishing tasks come to us automatically. We do them without thinking. Sometimes those habits serve us by saving us time and energy. We do not have to think about something; we just do it. Sometimes, however, that same process of doing things automatically leads us to continue to do things one way even though it may be problematic to do so.

The deadliest habits lead us to addictions and disorders. In these scenarios, we repeat the same behavior over and over again even if it eventually destroys us. It is what we know. It is what we know to do, and any other kind of behavior is uncomfortable or foreign to us.

Healthy habits, however, can lead to mental muscles. We do the right thing, the healthy thing, automatically, because that, too, is what we know and what we have practiced. Imagine that someone throws you a ball. If you are paying attention, you know exactly what to do. You follow the ball with your eyes, reach out, and grasp it as it comes to you. That process occurs easily because of the numerous opportunities we each have to practice the necessary skills in catching a ball. The same practice is necessary to develop healthy habits.

We learn healthy habits the same way that we learn unhealthy ones. Sometimes we learn things because two events co-occur. From Pavlov's (1927) classical conditioning paradigm, we can understand that we learn certain things reflexively, almost without our awareness. When studying the physiology of digestion, his classical experiment included placing meat powder in a dog's mouth. Salivation took place. Then some arbitrary stimulus, such as a light, was combined with the presentation of the meat powder. Finally, the light evoked salivation independent of the food. We may learn or acquire certain habits, then, simply because they co-occur with another event.

This process of learning can take on much significance when we think of events that co-occur in children's lives. For example, if dangerous or frightening things occur while a child is being held, the child can become frightened by human touch. Conversely, if being held co-occurs with a pleasant event, such as hearing a soothing voice, listening to a lullaby, or being fed, the child may enjoy being touched by others.

B. F. Skinner (1938) added further information and dimensions to help us understand how we learn behavior and shape our habits. In general, he said that we operate on our environment, and we are reinforced either positively or negatively for our behavior. We receive reinforcement and punishment constantly in our daily lives as responses to our behavior. If we receive positive reinforcement or reward, we are more likely to repeat the behavior. In most cases, however, punishment decreases the likelihood of a response recurring. It is interesting to note that reward or reinforcement is likely to increase a behavior and helps develop habitual behavior. Punishment, on the other hand, only seems to inhibit the expression of a behavior and may do nothing to help us develop healthy behavior.

The problems with punishment, particularly physical punishment, of children deserve special mention. For example, after a spanking, a child may be inhibited for a short period of time from performing a particular activity such as stealing or fighting; however, the response is only temporarily inhibited. When the child feels that there may not be any punishment for this action, he/she is likely to repeat it. Since physical discipline only has a temporary effect, it makes little sense to use it, especially when we know that it may encourage children to use physical methods themselves for solving their own problems.

Therefore, if we want to build healthy mental muscles in children through developing healthy habits, we first might consider two possibilities for decreasing unhealthy behavior: (a) we can ignore the negative or undesirable behavior as much as possible (Pransky, 1991) or (b) we can use some type of nonphysical punishment as a means to interrupt unhealthy behavior temporarily. Once interrupted, however, we need to focus more precisely on attending to good behavior and rewarding children positively for behaviors that promote a healthy way of living and relating. Positive rewards or reinforcements have much longer-lasting effects in helping shape children's behavior.

We might consider, then, that habits are ritualized ways of behaving that become integrated in the self and the in way we live. Habits can be constructive or destructive. Since the self is a physical, cognitive, emotional, spiritual, and social entity, we want to cultivate habits that develop each facet of the self in a constructive manner. These habits, then, become acquired skills in ways of living.

A more detailed look at habits that develop each facet of the self might be helpful. Healthy physical habits include building strong bodies through personal hygiene, balanced and nutritious diet, physical exercise, and adequate sleep and rest. Healthy cognitive habits include building a strong mind through acquiring an intellectual curiosity, a capacity to think for ourselves, a respect for our own thoughts, and an ability to learn from our own mistakes. Healthy emotional habits include building a strong psyche through acquiring skill to cope with personal emotions, acquiring ways to nurture the self, and acquiring resiliency to face difficult life situations. Healthy spiritual and social habits include building a strong, mutually valuing connectedness to the self, to the universe, and to other people.

During the elementary school years, children are still in a very formative stage in their habit development. They are especially open to adult reinforcement of positive, healthy behaviors. The elementary school years are a good time, then, to reach out to children with messages of positive reinforcement for those behaviors that promote personal and social competence.

We are creatures of habit. When our habits or rituals promote healthy ways of living and relating, we are developing traditions that exercise our mental muscles and build opportunities for life satisfaction. Our mental muscles grow stronger when we include traditions in our daily living that incorporate the many dimensions of ourselves and help us achieve balance. Balance, particularly between work and play, is a significant issue for elementary school children.

BALANCING WORK AND PLAY

To understand the importance of balance in our lives, we might think of the balance required in several physical endeavors. When balanced, these actions are beautiful. When out of balance, they lose their gracefulness and joy. A top spinning, a child riding a bicycle, a track star running the hurdles, an ice skater, a circus performer on the high wire all present beauty, grace, and productivity when in balance.

When we have balance in our personal lives, we provide ourselves with opportunities to enjoy a variety of different things, activities, and people. We also retain the likelihood that we will remain productive in each of these activities or areas.

Carl Jung (1961) emphasized the importance of balance to emotional and physical well-being. He stated that the psyche naturally attempts to achieve balance and a balanced system through seeking an equilibrium among the various aspects of the personality.

Each of us is complex. We need to balance a number of issues and priorities in our lives. As adults we must juggle multiple pressing needs and demands on us. We need to spend time with children, spouses, relatives, friends, and still have time alone. We need to work at our jobs, finish chores in our homes, and simply relax and play. We need to consider the needs and wishes of our own lives and the needs and wishes of others (Dlugokinski, 1990).

Children also are required to respond to many pressing needs and demands placed upon them. Even young children know that they need a balance between sleep and waking activity, a balance between being too cold and too hot, and a balance between stimulation and repose. Later, during the elementary school years, a major task for children is to develop a healthy work habit or a sense that they can work effectively and balance work with play in their lives (Erikson, 1968).

Balance is not achieved simply or quickly, but the early school years are the formative period where these important skills are learned. Parents, teachers, and other adult caregivers can provide the structure and framework for a healthy balanced work and play habit to develop. Adults can provide structure through a balance in schoolday activities, a consistent time and place for doing homework, and a list of chores with rewards for doing them. Furthermore, when children observe parents or other adults who balance work and play, this provides a powerful model for them.

It is easier for most children to play than it is to work. We need to motivate children to develop a healthy work habit. In order for a child to be motivated to work effectively, he/she must believe that some reward is waiting at the completion of the work task. For younger children, the reward needs to be more concrete and immediate. As children grow older, they are able to work for longer periods and sustain more hopes for later reinforcement (Moshman, Glover, & Bruning, 1987).

Children can enjoy more productive work if we can help them feel that their work is valued and meaningful. Each child needs to feel that their work can be appreciated. They need to know that they can offer a contribution to the larger community (Pransky, 1991). Perfection is not a goal. The idea is to encourage children to keep improving in their work (Glenn & Nelson, 1988). We can do this by creating a favorable work climate. In this climate, we help children make their work interesting and challenging and provide the opportunity for them to view themselves as competent and useful (Bevelle & Nickerson, 1981).

A 1992 survey of 28,000 workers found that people who feel least stressed at their jobs are those who have meaningful lives outside of work and those who have a chance to relax at the end of the day. A growing body of research shows that workers who strike a healthy balance between work, play, and family life are able to counter the negative effects of work burnout and stress (Custer, 1994). We need to help children develop this skill for balancing work and play in their lives, and we can begin this process in early childhood.

SUMMARY

Mental muscles provide children with strength, vigor, and stamina for living a healthy life. There are four ingredients that contribute to forming these muscles for elementary school children. First, children must learn that they have a right to develop a competent self. Second, children need to learn to respect this self and the selves of others by practicing personal and social responsibilities. Third, they need to develop strong, positive habits that can help the self ritualize healthy ways of living and relating. Finally, children need to find a balance between work and play for the self to feel useful and competent.

It is our community responsibility to help children acquire and exercise mental muscles that can help them lead satisfying and productive lives. In chapter 6 we have included lessons designed to build and exercise those muscles. We realize that these exercises provide only the framework for an educational process that needs to be practiced on a daily basis in children's lives. These exercises can be brought to life in daily practice when the community establishes clear priorities for the emotional development of children.

Chapter 6

PRACTICAL EXERCISES IN BUILDING MENTAL MUSCLES

These practical exercises were developed out of a need to give children practice in building strong and healthy resources for emotional resiliency. Some of the ideas in the exercises have been adapted from other curricula developed previously by the authors. Those curricula include the following: *I Am Special* (Allen & Dlugokinski, 1992); *The Secret of Work and Play* (Dlugokinski & Allen, 1994b); *Caring Connections* (Dlugokinski & Allen, 1991); and *Living in Self Esteem* (Dlugokinski & Allen, 1994a). The majority of the stories and exercises in this chapter are original, however, and have been created to help children build mental muscles through dedication and practice.

The suggested framework for delivering these exercises begins with a story and three introductory exercises. This story includes a song and an acronym for remembering the four mental muscles. Following the introductory exercises are four major sections of practical exercises. Each section emphasizes one of the mental muscles: Customs, Harmony, Esteem, and Wisdom. Major sections of the introductory story should be discussed with the children at the beginning of each of the four major sections, including singing the entire song at the beginning of each exercise. At the end of each exercise, we suggest singing the stanza that is particular to the section the children are studying.

Each theme section (Customs, Harmony, Esteem, Wisdom) is introduced with a vignette that highlights the particular mental muscle. This is followed by working definitions and a practice chart. The practice chart is included so that the major themes of each section can be practiced on a continuing basis. The charts are designed to call attention to healthy muscle formation in the children in each of the four areas. If the person who facilitates this program is not with the children on a daily basis, it is critical to engage someone who can carry out the activity of the chart.

INTRODUCTORY EXERCISES 1 THROUGH 3

Objective

To help children learn, integrate, and remember four ways that they can build mental muscles.

The following three exercises have been developed as an introduction to the Building Mental Muscles instruction program. They are designed to be used for both 5 through 7-year-olds and 8- through 11-year-olds.

INTRODUCTORY EXERCISE 1. TOM AND JERI ARE GROWING UP

Activity

Read or tell in detail the story, *Tom and Jeri Are Growing Up,* to the children. After completing the story, ask the children to recall with you major segments of the story. The song in the story, *So You Can Grow,* is put to music on an accompanying audiotape. Sheet music of the song is included as Figure 6.1. Play the song for the children after reading the story.

So You Can Grow

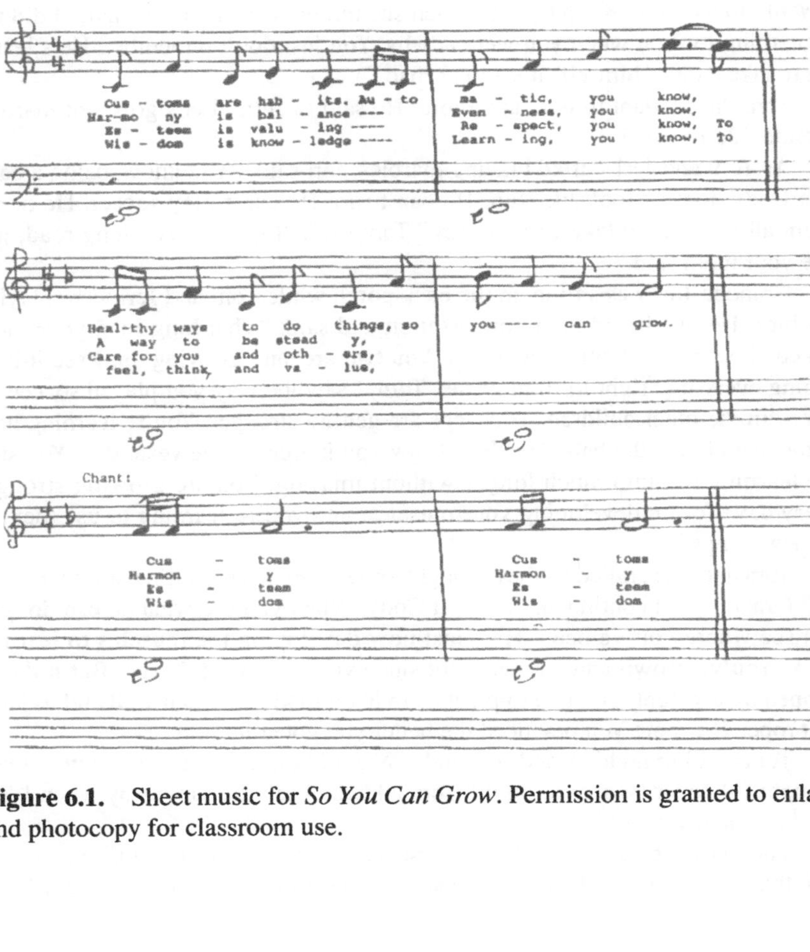

Figure 6.1. Sheet music for *So You Can Grow*. Permission is granted to enlarge and photocopy for classroom use.

Tom and Jeri Are Growing Up

One Saturday afternoon Tom and Jeri played soccer with several other children in the neighborhood. After they finished the game, they went to Jeri's house to play marbles. They were learning to take turns more often these days since Grandpa Jim had helped them with that.

As they walked into Jeri's house, they noticed her little brother, Cody. Cody was one year old and just starting to walk. He took a few good steps, then fell down and started to cry. Jeri went over to pick him up just as her mother walked in the room. Cody kept crying, so Jeri gave Cody to her mother.

Jeri's older sister, Sandra, came by and said "Oh, he's always crying. He didn't hurt himself. He always gets his way." Mom gave Cody a kiss on the cheek, patted him on the head, put him down on the floor, and said, "You'll learn to walk pretty soon. Keep trying." Then she turned to Sandra and said, "I did the same thing for you when you were a baby. You just don't remember. He's learning to take care of himself. It's a long road."

Tom didn't want to hear any more. He said to Jeri, "Let's go shoot marbles outside." Jeri agreed.

As Tom and Jeri started playing marbles, Jeri said, "You know, being a baby like Cody doesn't look like fun. He can't run. He can't play soccer. He needs Mom all the time to take care of him." Tom said, "I guess it *is* a long road, just like your mom said."

Grandpa Jim was sitting on the back porch while Tom and Jeri were playing marbles. He overheard their conversation and said, "That long road your mom talked about is all about growing up. You two are sure growing up. I see it happening every day right in front of me. Tom, I saw the way you played soccer today with the other children. Your legs are getting stronger. You're learning how to move and kick the ball. And Jeri, I saw you jumping rope yesterday. You sure are learning to jump much longer without missing. You are growing stronger every day. You're developing your muscles, and you're learning to use them to do new things."

Tom and Jeri smiled as they thought about themselves getting stronger.

Grandpa Jim continued, "Look at Cody. When you see what he can do, you can see where you've been. He's just now developing the muscles to learn to walk. You've grown and learned a lot since you were Cody's age. But it didn't happen by accident. You had to practice to learn to kick the ball well and to jump that rope. The more you practiced the better you got at it."

Tom and Jeri nodded, and Jeri said, "When I first started to try to jump rope I thought I'd never be able to do it." Tom added, "I felt the same way when I first tried to ride my bike."

Then Grandpa Jim said, "There are some other ways that you're growing, too, that aren't so easy to see. You can see your muscles building in your body, but you can't see muscles that are getting stronger inside your mind. My Grandmother Ruth used to say they were "Mental Muscles." She said mental muscles didn't grow by accident either. Building them takes practice and exercise. They help us take care of ourselves and live peacefully with others."

"Mental muscles?" Jeri said. "I've never heard of mental muscles." Both Tom and Jeri looked a bit puzzled.

Grandpa Jim walked over to a part of the garden where flowers were growing. He waved to Tom and Jeri to come join him. Grandpa Jim then bent down and dug up a little scrawny-looking yellow-leafed flower that looked like it was not growing very well. He dug it up carefully and placed it in a different place in the garden, about two feet away from where it was before.

Grandpa Jim then said to Tom and Jeri, "I wonder if you have any idea about why I put this flower in a new place in the garden." Tom said, "Maybe because it was sick, and it looked like it was dying." Grandpa Jim said, "Yes, but I want to know why you think it was dying."

Grandpa Jim then took Tom and Jeri over to the spot where he originally dug up the flower and said, "I want you to look at this spot for a minute and tell me what you see." Jeri said, "I see a big bush right next to where the flower used to be." Tom said, "Yes, and I see another bigger flower right in front of where you dug the hole." Grandpa Jim said, "Good, I think you're getting it." Tom and Jeri still looked a little puzzled. They said, "Well, what does that have to do with mental muscles?"

Grandpa Jim took Tom and Jeri back to the newly planted flower and said, "This flower needed its own place so it could grow. Tom and Jeri, each of you is like this flower. You need a place to grow and room to be your own person, just like the flower needs space to become beautiful. You need room to develop so you can learn to take care of yourself and live with others peacefully. If people try to do everything for you, they crowd you just like this flower, and you can't grow. Your parents and teachers can help, but you have to have your own space to grow because you are a separate person. This is the first step in building your mental muscles."

Both Tom and Jeri still looked a little puzzled. Then Tom asked, "You mean, when I was younger and my father made me learn to tie my own shoes, was that like giving me space to be a person?" "Exactly," said Grandpa Jim. Then Tom added, "I thought I'd never learn. I always wanted him to do it for me, but he said I had to learn to do it myself." Jeri said, "And my mom said that I had to brush my own hair every morning before school. At first I wanted her to do it for me, but now I fix my hair the way *I* like it." And Tom said, "Yeah, and I've learned to tie double knots in my shoes."

Grandpa Jim then said, "You've got it. You're understanding the first part about building mental muscles. Only *you* can learn to take care of yourself and get along with other people. No one can do it for you."

Then Grandpa Jim said, "I'd like to show you something that can help you learn and remember some things about mental muscles." Tom and Jeri looked interested.

Grandpa Jim said, "I want you to look at your hand. See how your thumb is separated from the rest of the fingers? It needs to be strong and separate from your fingers in order for your hand to work. Now, look at your four fingers. Just like you need all four fingers to make your hand strong, you need four strong mental muscles to make you a strong person."

As Grandpa Jim told Tom and Jeri each of the four things, he touched each of his four fingers. "You need to grow in customs, in harmony, in esteem, and in wisdom," he said. "Think of this word to help you remember the muscles you need—"CHEW." Just like you chew on food before you swallow it, you are going to have to chew on these ideas for quite a while before you understand what they mean."

Tom and Jeri said, "Chew?"

Grandpa Jim answered, "Yes." He touched his fingers one at a time again as he said, "C stands for customs, H for harmony, E for esteem, and W for wisdom."

Tom and Jeri said, "We don't know what those words mean. We don't understand them." Jeri said, "I don't know what you mean by harmony or wisdom." Tom chimed in, "And I don't know what the other two mean, esteem and customs."

Grandpa Jim said, "I'd like to sing a song that might help you understand what each of the words means." So Grandpa Jim sang:

So You Can Grow

Customs are habits,
Automatic, you know,
Healthy ways to do things,
So you can grow.
(Chant) Customs, Customs.

Harmony is balance,
Evenness, you know,
A way to be steady,
So you can grow.
(Chant) Harmony, Harmony.

Esteem is valuing,
Respect, you know,
To care for you and others,

So you can grow.
(Chant) Esteem, Esteem.

Wisdom is knowledge,
Learning, you know,
To feel, think, and value,
So you can grow.
(Chant) Wisdom, Wisdom.

Grandpa Jim sang the song again, this time with Tom and Jeri singing along with him. Then he said, "This is just the beginning of learning about these mental muscles. Maybe we'll talk about them one at a time so you can understand them better. But right now, sing the song. Chew on what those words might mean, and we'll talk later."

Grandpa Jim walked back into the house for a nap. Tom and Jeri went on playing marbles while they sang the song.

INTRODUCTORY EXERCISE 2. SO YOU CAN GROW

Activity

Review the major themes of the story, *Tom and Jeri Are Growing Up*. Consider having the children read the story themselves or role-play the story. Roles could include a narrator, Grandpa Jim, Tom, Jeri, Cody, Sandra, and Jeri's mother.

Use the last half of the session to teach the children the song *So You Can Grow*. Consider making copies of the sheet music (Figure 6.1) to help them remember the song.

Play the song (located on the accompanying audiotape) through once and have the children simply listen to the words and music. Play it through again, stopping after each verse, and have the children sing the verse with you. End the session by having the children sing through the entire song accompanied by the audiotaped version.

INTRODUCTORY EXERCISE 3. I CAN BUILD MENTAL MUSCLES

Activity

Review the story and sing the song. It would be helpful for the children to have a visual reminder of the four components of building mental muscles. One way to incorporate this reminder in a fun exercise is to have the children make their own poster, illustrating with their own artwork the four major components in building mental muscles. The poster could have this basic framework:

I CAN BUILD MENTAL MUSCLES

CUSTOMS

HARMONY

ESTEEM

WISDOM

PRACTICAL EXERCISES FOR CUSTOMS

Vignette (To Be Read with Customs Exercise 1)

One day Tom and Jeri were playing in the park near their house. Tom's mother came to the park and told him he had to go home and clean up his room. His mother told him to clean his room before he went out to play, but he forgot. Jeri heard Tom's mother say that Tom was grounded and could not come out for the rest of the day.

The next day, Tom and Jeri were shooting marbles, and Grandpa Jim overheard Tom say, "I just can't seem to get my room cleaned. I always forget, or when I remember, it always seems like there's something better to do."

Jeri said, "Yeah, I feel the same way about feeding the cat and changing the litter. I'm supposed to do it everyday, but whenever I think about the cat, I say I'll do it later. Then I get in trouble."

Grandpa Jim walked over with a rubber ball in his hand. He said to Tom and Jeri, "Watch this." Then he rolled the ball down the slope of the driveway.

Grandpa Jim then said, "Tom, Jeri, what did you notice about that ball?"

Tom said, "I noticed that it rolled slowly until it really started going down fast. It looked like it was easier for it to roll."

Jeri said, "It got in a groove and just kept rolling."

Grandpa Jim said, "Good, Tom. You need a groove, too, so you can make cleaning your room easier. Jeri, you need a groove to help you take care of the cat. A groove is like a habit or a custom. If you can get into the habit of doing these things at a certain time and place, it gets easier because you're used to doing it that way. You build a habit or custom for doing it a certain way at a certain time, and just like that ball rolling down the driveway, you roll easier—it gets easier because you're used to it."

Tom said, "What do you mean, build a custom? What's a custom?"

Grandpa Jim replied, "A custom is a regular way or time that you do something all the time. Once it gets regular, you don't have to think about it. It's a habit. It's what you're used to doing. For example, Tom, you have a customary time of eating with your family every evening at 5:30, and you know you have to be in bed by 8:30 on school nights. You're used to these ways of doing things. They are habits. They are customs. And Jeri, I know that you brush your teeth every morning after you eat. That's a custom, too. You do it regularly, just like clockwork. Those are customs that help you."

Grandpa Jim continued, "You also have customs or habits that may not help you. You've both gotten into a habit of saying 'I'll do it later' when it's time to clean your room or feed the cat. You both need a new custom. You need to think of a way to help you do it automatically, without thinking about it."

Tom and Jeri listened to Grandpa Jim's ideas. They thanked him and began playing marbles again. While they were playing, they talked about a way they might develop a custom so they could take care of their chores and stay out of trouble.

Working Definition

A ***custom*** is a habit; a regular or usual way that we do things, almost automatically, without thinking about it.

Practice Chart

Put the *Customs Practice Chart* (Figure 6.2) on the chalkboard. Use the chart to reinforce times when you notice children practicing healthy and unhealthy habits. Write the situation and child's name when you notice examples. When you notice an unhealthy habit, have the child and/or the class brainstorm about a new custom or habit they might develop instead of the troubling one.

CUSTOMS PRACTICE CHART

Healthy Customs/Habits		**Unhealthy Customs/Habits**		**What I Would Like as a New Custom**	
Name	Situation	Name	Situation	Name	Situation
Examples:		Example:		Example:	
John	Listening quietly to directions.	John	Interrupting without raising my hand.	John	Raising my hand before speaking
John	Beginning work immediately after the teacher assigns it.				

Figure 6.2. Customs Practice Chart.

CUSTOMS EXERCISE 1
(Ages 5 Through 7)

Objective

To help children understand the meaning of customs or habits, the importance of establishing healthy habits in their lives, and the importance of interrupting unhealthy habits.

Activity

Tell the children that Grandpa Jim is coming back to tell them more about mental muscles. Tell them that you want to read them another story about Grandpa Jim because he is going to give them some more information about another mental muscle called "customs."

Tell the children that you want them to listen carefully because you will ask them to tell you what happened in the story. Read the Customs Vignette to the children. With each section of the Customs Vignette, ask the children to recall what happened next.

Ask the children, "What do you think it means to have customs or habits in your life?"

After the children have given you their ideas, tell them that custom means a habit, a regular or usual way of doing things, almost automatically, without thinking about it.

Tell the children that Grandpa Jim knows how to have healthy customs or habits in his life. Ask them if they know why. Accept several answers.

Now tell the children that Grandpa Jim learned a lot about customs or habits as a way of taking care of himself from Grandmother Ruth. Then he practiced what he learned.

Tell the children that in the rest of the exercises on customs, they will learn more about how to have healthy customs or habits in their own lives.

CUSTOMS EXERCISES 2, 3, AND 4 (Ages 5 Through 7)

Activity

The following format is to be used for Exercises 2, 3, and 4. In Exercise 2, focus on habits at school; in Exercise 3, habits at home; and in Exercise 4, habits in the neighborhood or general community.

1. Tell the children that you want them to think with you about the habits they have now. Remind them that Grandpa Jim told them that they can have habits that can help them or habits that can hurt them.
2. Ask the children to tell you about habits they feel can be helpful at school. Try to accept at least 12 to 15 responses and list them on the board.
3. Take volunteers who think they can demonstrate (role-play) how these healthy habits look for the rest of the class. An example is as follows:
   In school, a healthy habit would be sitting quietly and listening to directions and raising your hand before speaking.
4. Identify habits that the children think are harmful and list those on the board.
5. Tell the children that habits that are harmful to us sometimes occur almost automatically, but we can stop those habits by telling ourselves to STOP and then doing something else instead.
6. Ask for volunteers who will demonstrate this technique with various harmful situations listed on the chalkboard. Have the children role-play the STOP procedure and then role-play what they would like as a new habit.

CUSTOMS EXERCISE 5
(Ages 5 Through 7)

Materials

- Provide a photocopy of the *Stop and Go with Customs* page (Figure 6.3) for each child.
- Crayons

Activity

Ask the children to look with you at the *Stop and Go with Customs* page (Figure 6.3).

Tell the children that the picture they are looking at is a stoplight. In the top circle, you want them to write about or draw a picture of a habit they want to stop. In the bottom circle, you want them to write or draw a habit they want to develop or increase. In the middle circle, have the children write their name. Finally, lightly color the three circles: top-red; middle-yellow; bottom-green. Ask the children to color lightly enough that their writing or drawing can be seen. Finish with a discussion and allow children to share with the class what they wrote or drew on the stoplight.

STOP AND GO WITH CUSTOMS (HABITS)

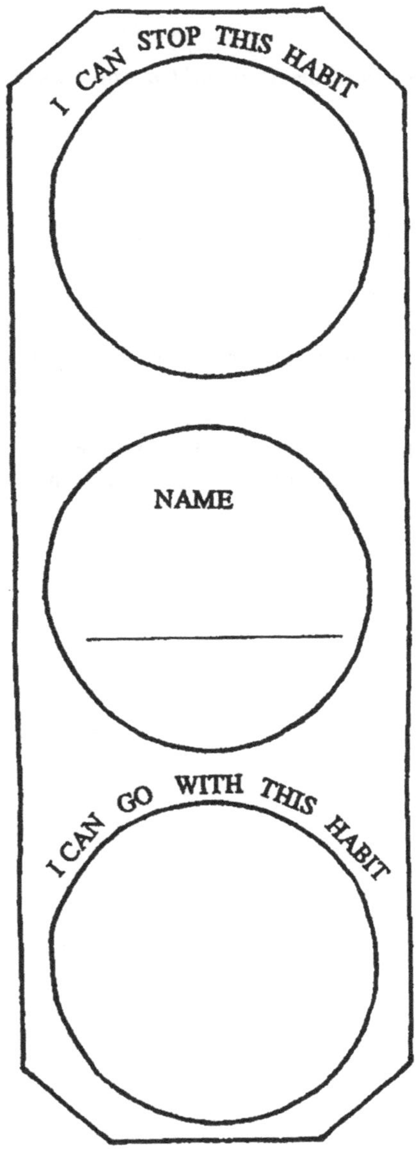

Figure 6.3. Stop and Go with Customs (Habits). Permission is granted to enlarge and photocopy for classroom use.

CUSTOMS EXERCISE 1
(Ages 8 Through 11)

Objective

To help children understand the meaning of customs or habits, the importance of establishing healthy habits in their lives, and the importance of interrupting unhealthy habits.

Activity

Tell the children that Grandpa Jim is coming back to tell them more about mental muscles. Tell them that you want to read them another story about Grandpa Jim because he is going to give them some more information about another mental muscle called "customs."

Tell the children that you want them to listen carefully because you will ask them to tell you what happened in the story. Read the Customs Vignette to the children. With each section of the Customs Vignette, ask the children to recall what happened next.

Ask the children, "What do you think it means to have customs or habits in your life?"

After the children have given you their ideas, tell them that custom means a habit, a regular or usual way of doing things, almost automatically, without thinking about it.

Tell the children that Grandpa Jim knows how to have healthy customs or habits in his life. Ask them if they know why. Accept several answers.

Now tell the children that Grandpa Jim learned a lot about customs or habits as a way of taking care of himself from Grandmother Ruth. Then he practiced what he learned.

Tell the children that in the rest of the exercises on customs, they will learn more about how to have healthy customs or habits in their own lives.

CUSTOMS EXERCISE 2
(Ages 8 Through 11)

Materials

Provide each child with a photocopy of the *I Can Change My Customs (Habits)* page (Figure 6.4).

Activity

Tell the children that you want them to think with you about the habits they have now. Remind them that Grandpa Jim told them that they can have healthy habits that can help them or unhealthy habits that can hurt them.

Write three categories on the chalkboard: Home, School, Neighborhood. Have the children brainstorm with you and identify 10 unhealthy habits they can have in each of these categories.

Repeat the above procedure, only this time identify healthy habits.

Now ask the children to choose from the list one healthy habit they would like to develop and one unhealthy habit they would like to eliminate. Ask them to write these habits in the appropriate space on the *I Can Change My Customs (Habits)* page (Figure 6.4).

I CAN CHANGE MY CUSTOMS (HABITS)

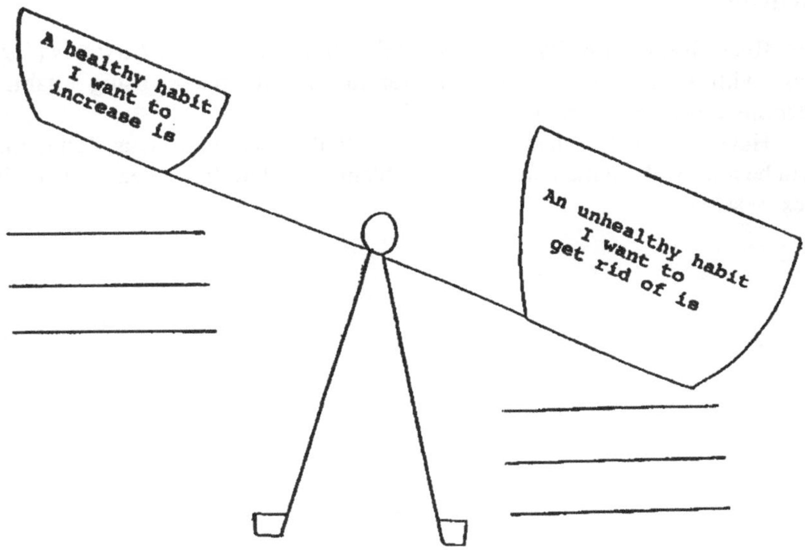

Figure 6.4. I Can Change My Customs (Habits). Permission is granted to enlarge and photocopy for classroom use.

CUSTOMS EXERCISE 3
(Ages 8 Through 11)

Materials

Provide a photocopy of the *Planning Sheet for Building Healthy Customs (Habits)* page (Figure 6.5) for each child.

Activity

Read through the *Planning Sheet for Building Healthy Customs (Habits)* page with the children. Ask the children to fill in the blanks using a habit they identified that they wanted to build in Exercise 2.

Have the children share and discuss with the class their plans. Tell them you will be asking about their success or problems with building a healthy habit in the next session.

Planning Sheet
for Building Healthy Customs (Habits)

1. Identify the habit you want to develop. ______________________
2. Identify the specific day(s) and time(s) you will begin practicing this habit. ______________________________________

Examples:

- Every morning right after breakfast I will feed the dog.
- Every Thursday evening beginning at 7:00 I will clean my room. I will try to have it done by 7:30.

Days I will practice my habit are ______________________________
____.

Times I will practice my habit are _____________________________
____.

3. This is what I will tell myself when the job is done:
   ____
   ____
   ____.

Figure 6.5. Planning Sheet for Building Healthy Customs (Habits). Permission is granted to enlarge and photocopy for classroom use.

CUSTOMS EXERCISE 4
(Ages 8 Through 11)

Materials

Provide a photocopy of the *Planning Sheet for Overcoming an Unhealthy Custom (Habit)* page (Figure 6.6) for each child.

Activity

Begin with a discussion of the children's successes and problems in their plan from the previous week to increase a healthy habit.

Read through the *Planning Sheet for Overcoming an Unhealthy Custom (Habit)* page with the children. Ask the children to fill in the blanks.

Have the children share and discuss with the class their plans. Tell them you will be asking about their success or problems with their plan in the next session.

Planning Sheet
for Overcoming an Unhealthy Custom (Habit)

1. Identify the unhealthy habit you want to overcome:

   ____.

2. How much effort are you willing to put toward overcoming this unhealthy habit? Circle the number below that answers this question.

1	2	3	4	5
A little effort				A lot of effort

3. What hint can you give yourself to help you remember that you want to stop this habit? ____

   ____

Examples:

- I can put a note to myself on my desk that says: No fighting; no walking around in the classroom, etc.
- I can draw a picture with an X through it of what I don't want to do.
- I can wear a rubber band on my wrist to remind me.

4. List some things you can do instead of your unhealthy habit: ________

   ____

   ____

Examples:

- Instead of fighting, I could put my hands in my pocket and walk away.
- Instead of bossing my friend around, I could find something nice to say about my friend or ask him/her what he/she would like to do.

5. Write something you will say to yourself if you are able to break your bad habit: ________________________________

____

____

____

Examples:

- I did a good job.
- I'm proud of me for overcoming a bad habit.

Figure 6.6. Planning Sheet for Overcoming an Unhealthy Custom (Habit). Permission is granted to enlarge and photocopy for classroom use.

CUSTOMS EXERCISE 5
(Ages 8 Through 11)

Materials

- Butcher paper or poster boards
- Magic markers, crayons, or painting supplies

Activity

This activity may take more than one session to achieve its fullest benefit. Tell the children that one way people are reminded to overcome unhealthy habits and build healthy ones is through media campaigns.

Discuss with the children some habits they think are most healthy for their school or community to develop. List those on the board.

Repeat the above procedure, only this time list unhealthy habits.

Divide the class into groups of 3 or 4 children each. Have each group design a poster (e.g., picture and slogan) depicting either a healthy habit they would like themselves and others to adopt or an unhealthy habit they would like themselves and others to overcome. Tell the group to

1. Identify the habit.
2. Brainstorm together to come up with a slogan.
3. Brainstorm together to come up with ideas for a picture.
4. Decide what role each group member can have in finishing the poster.
5. Finish the poster.

Have the children share and discuss their posters with the class. If possible, allow them to share their posters and ideas with other classrooms.

PRACTICAL EXERCISES FOR HARMONY

Vignette (To Be Read with Harmony Exercise 1)

Tom and Jeri had become very good friends. In fact, they enjoyed playing together so much that sometimes they didn't want to stop playing. They didn't want to come inside after recess was over, do their work at school, or do their chores at home. At school, their grades were beginning to go down. At home, their rooms were a mess. Their parents nagged at them all the time to do their chores. Their teacher, Mrs. Turner, even called their parents at home and said she was worried about them.

Grandpa Jim was working in the garden. He heard Tom and Jeri say that they wanted to do well at school and home, but they really didn't want to give up having fun. Then Grandpa Jim came over to the two children, and he was holding something in his hand. He said to them, "I want you to watch this top spin." Then Grandpa Jim spun the top for the children on the patio. It stayed upright for about 30 seconds and then fell over.

Grandpa Jim asked the children, "Why do you think the top was able to spin?" Tom and Jeri said, "Because it was going fast." Grandpa Jim said, "Yes, that's true, but there's another reason. It's the same reason that it stopped and fell over." Then Tom said, "Oh, 'cause it's balanced." "Very good, Tom," Grandpa Jim replied.

Then Grandpa Jim said, "You're a little bit like this top." The children looked a bit puzzled. "Like the top?" Jeri asked.

"Yes," said Grandpa Jim. "When you have balance and harmony in your life, you run smoothly, just like the top does. When you don't, you'll fall down."

Grandpa Jim continued, "I heard both of you talking about how you like to play all the time. Playing is fun, but work and play are both important. You need them both to help you grow. Work is not as easy as play, but work helps you take care of yourself."

Tom said, "I *could* enjoy playing more if my parents didn't nag me all the time about my chores." Jeri added, "I don't feel too good when I get behind in my work at school, either."

Grandpa Jim said, "Balance in work and play is important. When you've got work to do, get started right away. You need a harmony or balance with a lot of things in your life, just like the top, so you can run well."

"What other things?" asked Jeri.

Then Grandpa Jim added, "Well, harmony is like a pleasant combination of things. Just like you need work and play, you need to sleep and be awake. You need to spend time with your friends and time by yourself. You need time at school and time at home. You need food, but a balance of the right kinds of food. Too much or not enough of any one thing—play, work, food, sleep, or even tele-

Too much or not enough of any one thing—play, work, food, sleep, or even television, can lead to trouble.

"Just like a cold glass of water tastes good when you've been hot and dry for a while, balance in all of these things is what helps you enjoy them. Finding a balance between work and play, and rest and activity is part of the secret to building strong mental muscles."

Grandpa Jim went back and sat down on the porch. Both Tom and Jeri thought about that top spinning for a long time. They remembered the top and the balance that Grandpa Jim talked about when they had work to do. Work still wasn't as easy as play but they seemed to get to it better and get it done. Then their play was even more fun. Sometimes, too, after they watched television for a long time, they turned it off and found something else to do. They discovered that harmony and balance were important and helped them enjoy their life more.

Working Definition

Harmony is a balance between things that are opposites. A pleasant or comfortable combination of things that allows us to enjoy our life and function effectively.

Practice Chart

Put the *Harmony Practice Chart* (Figure 6.7) on the chalkboard. Use the chart to reinforce times when the children are shifting activities in order to achieve a balance or harmony in their daily schedule (e.g., recess after classwork, working alone and working with the whole class, eating a balanced lunch, resting after running, etc.). Write the situations that bring harmony and the child or children's name when you notice a good example of harmony or balance.

HARMONY PRACTICE CHART

Situations That Bring Harmony	Child/Children's Name(s)

Figure 6.7. Harmony Practice Chart.

HARMONY EXERCISE 1
(Ages 5 Through 7)

Objective

To help children understand the meaning of harmony or balance and the importance of achieving balance in their daily activities.

Activity

Tell the children that Grandpa Jim is coming back to tell them more about mental muscles. Tell them that you want to read them another story about Grandpa Jim because he is going to give them some more information about another mental muscle called harmony.

Tell the children that you want them to listen carefully because you will ask them to tell you what happened in the story.

Read the Harmony Vignette (located at the beginning of the harmony section of this chapter) to the children. Now, with each section of the vignette, ask the children to recall what happened next.

Ask the children, "What do you think it means to have harmony or balance in your life?"

After the children have given you their ideas, tell them that harmony means having a balance between things that are opposites. It is a pleasant or comfortable combination of things that allows us to enjoy our life and do things well."

Tell the children that Grandpa Jim knows how to have harmony or balance in his life. Ask them if they know why. Accept several answers.

Now tell the children that Grandpa Jim learned a lot about harmony or balance as a way of taking care of himself from Grandmother Ruth. Then he practiced what he learned.

Tell the children that in the rest of the exercises on harmony, they will learn more about how to have harmony or balance in their own lives.

HARMONY EXERCISE 2
(Ages 5 Through 7)

Procedure for Harmony Exercises 2, 3, 4, and 5

For Exercises 2, 3, 4, and 5, lead the children through the "action and relaxation" or "work and play" contrasting activities below. Then discuss with the children the activities in the following sequence:

1. Their experience with "action" or "work." What felt pleasant and/or unpleasant about it?
2. Their experience "relaxation" or "play." What felt pleasant or unpleasant about it?
3. Help the children notice the contrast between action and relaxation or work and play and the need for balance between the two. Help them notice that the contrast between the two helps them enjoy both and helps them build mental muscles.
4. Ask the children to discuss which of the contrasting activities, action and relaxation or work and play, they would need more of to have more balance or harmony in their life.
5. If time remains, have the children fold an 8-1/2" x 11" piece of paper in half. Ask them to draw "action" or "work" on one half of the paper and "relaxation" or "play on the other half. If they can write, ask them to write the following at the top of the page: I NEED BOTH OF THESE FOR HARMONY.

Contrasting Activities #1 and #2—Action and Relaxation

Action: Have the children stand up and run in place beside their desk for approximately one minute.

Relaxation: Have the children sit down, relax, and remain still and silent for one minute.

Action: Have the children make a fist with both hands. Ask them to squeeze very tightly for 30 seconds.

Relaxation: Tell the children to open their fists and relax their hand, palms open, fingers outstretched.

Action: Have the children hold their arms and hands stretched out parallel to their shoulders, with their palms facing upwards, as straight as they can.

Relaxation: Ask the children to return their arms to their side and rest them, arms and hands limp and relaxed.

HARMONY EXERCISE 3
(Ages 5 Through 7)

Contrasting Activity #1—Work

Materials.

- 1 small jar for each child (a baby food jar is about right)
- Chilled whipping cream (enough for each child to have 1/3 of a baby food jar of cream)
- Yellow food coloring (if desired for yellowed butter)
- 1 craft stick (lollipop stick) per child
- Crackers
- Jelly
- Blunt knife for spreading jelly
- Paper towels on which to serve crackers, butter, and jelly

Procedure. Tell the children that they are going to assist you in making something today. Tell them that you *and* they will work together to make something to eat, and then the class can enjoy sampling what they have made.

Tell the children that butter is made from cream and that they will be making their own butter. After they have worked hard to make the butter, they will be allowed to spread it on crackers and have a snack of crackers, butter, and jelly.

Give each of the children a baby food jar. Fill the jars one-third full of whipping cream. Put the tops on the jars tightly and ask the children to shake their jars until butter forms. Tell them that making the butter is not easy, but eating the butter and sharing the work and a snack with friends can be a very enjoyable experience.

Check the children's jars every few minutes. When butter has formed and most of the liquid is gone, drain the liquid off, put in one drop of yellow food coloring (if desired), and give each child a craft stick (popsicle stick) to stir food coloring into the butter.

Contrasting Activity #2—Play

Give the children two crackers. Allow them to spread the butter on the crackers with their craft stick. Add jelly, if desired, eat their snack, and enjoy.

Talk to the children about the work experience. Make the following points:

1. Work is not easy.
2. When shared with a friend, it sometimes can be more enjoyable.
3. After work is done, it is pleasant to enjoy what you've done. You can feel proud that you've done it.
4. Sometimes what you've worked on can be eaten, sometimes worn, sometimes simply looked at and enjoyed.

HARMONY EXERCISE 4
(Ages 5 Through 7)

Contrasting Activity #1—Work

Have the children clean out their desks or tables and wash off the tops with paper towels. Also ask them to clean the general classroom area. Tell them that, if they can do a good job, they will have an extra 10-minute recess.

Contrasting Activity #2—Play

Allow the children to go outside and play for 10 minutes, if weather permits. If not, give them a 10-minute quiet play time in the classroom.

HARMONY EXERCISE 5
(Ages 5 Through 7)

Contrasting Activity #1—Work

Materials.

- 5 plastic trash bags

Procedure. Tell the children that today they are going outside to work with their bodies, and you will be working with them. Choose a specific area of the playground for the class to pick up trash and litter and place it in trash bags. Choose an area that can be easily picked up by 25 children who are outside for 10 minutes.

Tell the children that this activity is a cooperative project. The children will be placed in groups of five. One child will hold the trash bag while the other four pick up pieces of trash or litter and put them in the bag. Emphasize to the children that they can get more done and enjoy the activity more if they try to help themselves and one another by doing their fair share of the work.

Place the children in groups of five. Assign one child per group to hold the trash bag for the group. Tell the children that it is important to remember who is holding the bag for their group.

Take the children outside to the designated playground area. Ask the children to look at the playground area to be picked up and describe to you what they see that they will be placing in their trash bags. Allow them to pick up litter or trash for 10 minutes.

Contrasting Activity #2—Play

Allow the children to play outside and enjoy the space they have picked up.

HARMONY EXERCISE 1
(Ages 8 Through 11)

Objective

To help children understand the meaning of harmony or balance and the importance of achieving balance in their daily activities.

Activity

Tell the children that Grandpa Jim is coming back to tell them more about mental muscles. Tell them that you want to read them another story about Grandpa Jim because he is going to give them some more information about another mental muscle called harmony.

Tell the children that you want them to listen carefully because you will ask them to tell you what happened in the story.

Read the Harmony Vignette (located at the beginning of the harmony section of this chapter) to the children. Now, with each section of the vignette, ask the children to recall what happened next.

Ask the children, "What do you think it means to have harmony or balance in your life?"

After the children have given you their ideas, tell them that harmony means having a balance between things that are opposites. It is a pleasant or comfortable combination of things that allows us to enjoy our life and do things well."

Tell the children that Grandpa Jim knows how to have harmony or balance in his life. Ask them if they know why. Accept several answers.

Now tell the children that Grandpa Jim learned a lot about harmony or balance as a way of taking care of himself from Grandmother Ruth. Then he practiced what he learned.

Tell the children that in the rest of the exercises on harmony, they will learn more about how to have harmony or balance in their own lives.

HARMONY EXERCISE 2
(Ages 8 Through 11)

Activity

Tell the children that sometimes it is difficult to achieve balance because some activities feel more difficult to do. Give the children some examples of activities that may be difficult to initiate. Examples are as follows:

going to bed on time,
eating a balanced diet,
doing chores at home,
getting started on work assignments in class, and
turning off the television or video game.

Write these and additional examples that the children give you on the chalkboard. Then, with each item, where difficulty is noted, have the children decide

1. a first step in getting this activity done, a small thing they could do to get started and
2. a reward or contrasting activity they could give themselves when they complete the task.

Have each child choose one of the activities that he/she thinks will be most difficult and a reward that he/she will choose to practice this week.

Ask the children to draw a picture of the activity and the reward and tell them that you want them to practice that activity this week.

HARMONY EXERCISE 3
(Ages 8 Through 11)

Activity

Ask the children to share with you their experiences from the past week in doing the difficult activity they chose.

Ask the children, "What rewards were given?" "What felt successful in the experience?" "What was difficult about the experience?" "Did anyone complete the task and reward themselves?"

For those children who experienced difficulty, have the class brainstorm together about things they might do or say to help themselves complete their task.

Ask for volunteers who are willing to pantomime or role-play in front of the class the steps involved in doing their difficult activity and reward.

HARMONY EXERCISE 4
(Ages 8 Through 11)

Activity

Tell the children that distractions sometimes make it harder to get work done. Tell them that distractions are things going on inside of us or outside of us that keep our attention off our work.

Engage the children to list with you the kinds of distractions they face in getting their schoolwork done or chores done at home. List them on the chalkboard under the categories given below.

Inside Distractions	Example: Thinking about program I'm going to watch.	Example: I'm upset because I can't go outside.
Outside Distractions	Example: Somebody is whispering to me.	Example: The kids are knocking on the door and saying come outside.

After several distractions are listed on the chalkboard, have the children brainstorm about something they could do or say to themselves that might help them finish the job they need to do.

Have the children role-play several examples of tasks they might be doing, with another child trying to distract them from the task. Have the child who is role-playing the task do something or say something that respectfully deals with the distraction, so they can get back to the task.

Tell the children that you want them to practice this week dealing with distractions so they can complete their work. If they are successful, remind them that they can reward themselves with an enjoyable experience.

HARMONY EXERCISE 5
(Ages 8 Through 11)

Materials

Provide each child with a photocopy *My Mandala for Balance* (Figure 6.8).

Activity

Tell the children that a mandala is a symbol of a balanced person and that they are going to create a mandala today.

As you look at the mandala with the children, describe each of the contrasting elements.

Have the children draw or write in their own activity that fits each of the separate sections. Children can also color the sections as they choose. The same color might be used for contrasting elements (e.g., work and play). As time permits, have children share their mandalas with each other and discuss the different activities they have chosen.

Conclude with a discussion of how balance builds mental muscles.

MY MANDALA FOR BALANCE

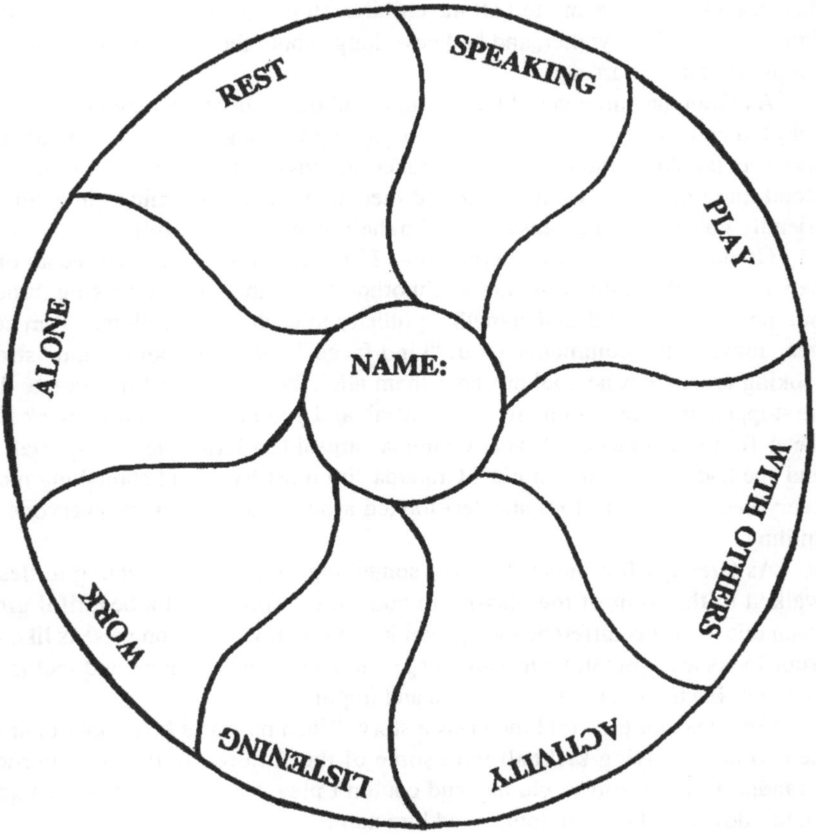

Figure 6.8. My Mandala for Balance. Permission is granted to enlarge and photocopy for classroom use.

PRACTICAL EXERCISES FOR ESTEEM

Vignette (To Be Read with Esteem Exercise 1)

One day Grandpa Jim visited Tom and Jeri at school. He had been invited by their teacher to come and tell all the children stories about growing up. Grandpa Jim was a good storyteller, and he knew things about the land and their town that happened many years ago.

As Grandpa Jim entered the room, the children became very quiet. He was very tall and so very impressive, with a greying face and kind eyes. Grandpa Jim was special. After the teacher introduced the visitor to the class, Grandpa Jim stood there quietly for a moment and then said, "Good morning" in a soft and friendly voice. The class answered with their own "Good morning."

Grandpa Jim then said, "Every year, I visit classrooms so I can see all of the new faces of the children in our neighborhood." He then began walking throughout the classroom and said something quietly to each of the children. Tom could hear some of the comments about "kind faces," "pretty ribbons," and "strong-looking arms," but he couldn't hear them all. When Grandpa Jim came to Tom, he stopped and said, "You are very special, and you have nice, curly black hair." Then Tom heard pieces of what Grandpa Jim said to Jeri—she was special, too, and she had a "very nice smile." Grandpa Jim must have said something nice to everyone, because as Tom and Jeri looked around the classroom, everyone was smiling.

As Grandpa Jim finished saying something to each of the young turtles, he walked to the front of the classroom and said, "You are all a beautiful group. Each one of you is different and special in your own way. No one else is like you. Your looks are special, your walk is special, and what you think and feel is special, too. Each one of you is valuable and important."

Grandpa Jim then told the class a story. When he was a boy about their age, he had been playing kickball with some of the children in the neighborhood. Grandpa Jim was sort of clumsy and couldn't play very well. During this game, he fell down, and the children called him names.

He then said, "I went home, and as I walked in the door, I was almost crying when I said to my Grandmother Ruth, 'I can't do anything right. The children are all making fun of me. I'm not worth anything.' Then I ran off to my room. Grandmother Ruth knew that I was very upset and wasn't in the mood to listen or talk, but later, after supper time, she said she wanted to talk with me."

"We sat down on the sofa together, and Grandmother Ruth gave me a glass of milk and a warm cookie. Then she said, 'Jim, I know how upset you were this afternoon when things didn't go well at the kickball game. It's no fun when kids make fun of you. I just want you to know that I love you just the way you are. You are valuable and special. In fact, everyone in this world is special and valuable in their own way.' Grandmother Ruth continued, 'I always want you to remember that you are good enough and that you deserve love and kindness. That means that you deserve to esteem yourself. Other people deserve esteem too, because we are all valuable. None of us is perfect, and we don't have to be. All of us deserve esteem.'"

Grandpa Jim then said, "I've always remembered the warm feeling I had inside when Grandmother Ruth told me this. Later, when the children called me names again, I tried to remember that warm feeling and not pay attention to what they said. Now Grandmother Ruth is giving you the same message through me. You are all very special, very valuable, and deserve esteem just the way you are."

Working Definition

To ***esteem*** is to honor, value, respect, cherish, hold in high regard—to treat in a special and positive way.

Practice Chart

Make a larger version of the *Esteem Practice Chart* (Figure 6.9). The chart should be large enough to be seen by children in a classroom setting.

Children need practice and exercise to develop strong mental muscles. The chart will be used as a reminder and reinforcement to the children of times when they are esteeming themselves and others.

Look for times during the week when feelings are owned and expressed constructively, when thoughts are used in a helpful way, and/or when someone has acted in a respectful way to self and others.

Put names and incidents on the practice chart. Keep adding to the lists, praising children for expressing feelings and thinking constructively, and for acting in a way that esteems themselves and others.

ESTEEM PRACTICE CHART

I value myself and others by . . .

Expressing feelings constructively		Using my thoughts in a helpful way		Acting in a way that is respectful to self and othersy	
Name	Incident	Name	Incident	Name	Incident

Figure 6.9. Esteem Practice Chart.

ESTEEM EXERCISE 1
(Ages 5 Through 7)

Objective

To help children understand the meaning of esteem and ways to respect and care for themselves and others simultaneously.

Activity

Tell the children that Grandpa Jim is coming back to tell them more about mental muscles. Tell them that you want to read them another story about Grandpa Jim because he is going to give them some more information about another mental muscle called esteem.

Tell the children that you want them to listen carefully because you will ask them to tell you what happened in the story.

Read the Esteem Vignette to the children located at the beginning of the Esteem section. Now, with each section of the vignette, ask the children to recall what happened next.

Ask the children, "What do you think it means to have esteem or to esteem yourself and others?"

After the children have given you their ideas, tell them that esteem means "that you treat yourself and others like valuable persons, with kindness and respect."

Tell the children that Grandpa Jim knows how to esteem himself and others. Ask them if they know why. Accept several answers.

Now tell the children that Grandpa Jim learned a lot about esteeming or taking care of himself and respecting others from Grandmother Ruth. Then he practiced what he learned.

Tell the children that in the rest of the exercises on esteem, they will learn more about treating themselves and others kindly, with respect.

ESTEEM EXERCISE 2
(Ages 5 Through 7)

Materials

- A photocopy of *I Am Special* (Figure 6.10) should be provided for each child.
- Tape measure
- Pencil and crayons

Activity

Remind the children that in the last exercise Grandpa Jim told Tom and Jeri and their friends that they were special, valuable, and deserving of respect and esteem.

Ask the children if they can remember what esteem means. Accept several answers, then review the definition of esteem located under Working Definition.

Ask the children to look with you at the *I Am Special* page (Figure 6.10). Help each child fill in the information required. Some children may have difficulty describing their own color of eyes or hair color, so they might be assigned a partner to help describe themselves. Also, in measuring height, adult assistance may be required for each child. Ask each child to draw a picture of himself/herself on the right hand side of the worksheet. If time permits, allow the children to color their "self" pictures.

Tell the children that one way they can esteem themselves is to remember that they are special.

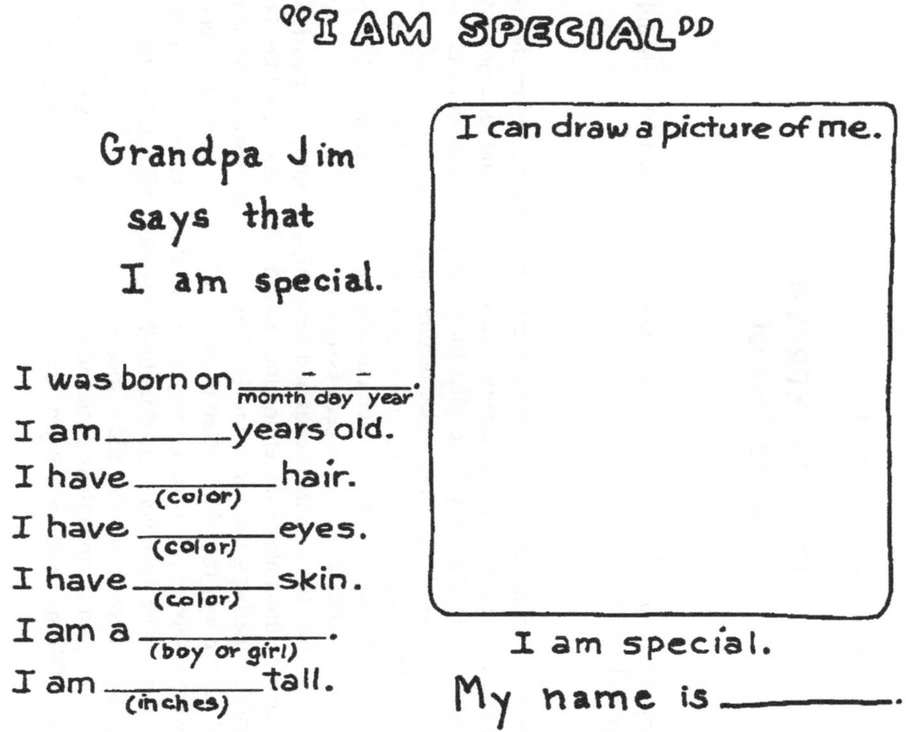

Figure 6.10. I Am Special. Permission is granted to enlarge and photocopy for classroom use.

ESTEEM EXERCISE 3
(Ages 5 Through 7)

Materials

A photocopy of *You Are Special* (Figure 6.11) should be provided for each child.
Crayons for each child

Activity

Review with the children the meaning of esteem. Tell the children that one way they can esteem themselves and others is through giving and receiving gifts.

Tell the children that they have gifts they can give to others—perhaps through using kind words, drawing a nice picture for a friend, or helping someone. Tell them that today the class is going to give and receive gifts.

Assign another child's name to each child in the class. Tell each child privately which child's name he/she has been assigned.

Ask the children to close their eyes and each think about his/her assigned child. Ask them to think about something they have noticed that they like about the other child . . . perhaps it is something they have seen this person doing on the playground . . . the way this child talked to other children . . . a special talent or ability they have noticed . . . a special way the other child combs his/her hair or dresses . . . or the way the other child does his/her work at school. Ask the children each to think about how this child is special.

Ask the children to open their eyes and look at the *You Are Special* page (Figure 6.11). Tell the children that you want them to color the picture on the page.

After the children have finished coloring, ask four or five children at a time to find their assigned classmate and give them their gift (i.e., balloon picture on page), and ask each child to tell his/her assigned classmate what he/she thinks is special about the person receiving the gift.

Ask the children to share their thoughts and feelings about giving these gifts to each other.

You Are Special

NAME ______________________________

Assigned Classmate ______________________________

One way you are special is ______________________________

Here is a special picture I have colored for you.

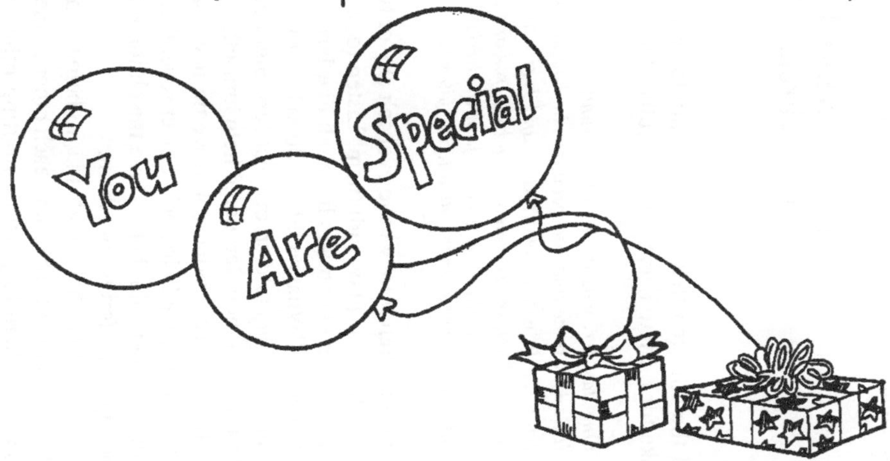

Figure 6.11. You Are Special. Permission is granted to enlarge and photocopy for classroom use.

ESTEEM EXERCISE 4
(Ages 5 Through 7)

Activity

Tell the children that you are going to read a story to them and that you would like for them to listen very carefully. Read the following story:

> *One day Jeri was on the playground at recess. She was feeling a little lonesome and sad because she had no one to play with. Her friend, Jill, was absent today, and Jeri was standing around by herself. Then shė slumped down by a tree and started to pick at the grass. She wanted to go and join in the kickball game with the other girls, but she was afraid. She felt shy.*

Ask the children if they have ever felt shy or timid—like they were afraid to ask other children to play with them. Listen to several examples from the children of times when they might have felt like Jeri.

Ask the class, "What could Jeri do to help or esteem herself?" Accept several suggestions from the children of what Jeri might do. Have the children role-play several examples of how Jeri could help himself.

Ask the children, "What could we do if we saw Jeri on the playground by herself? How could we help her?" Select several examples from children of how they might have her join them. Have the children role-play several examples of how they might ask Jeri to join them.

Tell the children that we all like to belong and feel like we are part of the group. We can help ourselves and each other to make friends. Tell them that this week you want them to practice inviting others to join them as they play in groups.

ESTEEM EXERCISE 5
(Ages 5 Through 7)

Materials

- A photocopy of *I Can Learn to Share* (Figure 6.12) should be provided for each child.
- Crayons for each child

Activity

Read the following story to the children:

> *One day Tom's Uncle John and Tom's cousin Jack came to visit at Tom's house. His Uncle John bought Tom and Jack a kite for both of them to play with. They went outside and started to play with the kite. Tom held the kite and helped it get up, and Jack held the string. After the kite went up, Tom wanted to have a turn to hold the kite, but Jack wouldn't let him. Jack said it was his kite and Tom couldn't hold it.*

Lead the class in a discussion: Was Jack being fair with Tom? Why or why not? (Try to bring out the idea that friends need to share with each other and take turns.)

Ask the children, "Why do you think Jack was unwilling to share?" (Elicit several responses of possible reasons he did not share and try to bring out the notion that sometimes it is not easy to share. We want to do things ourselves or we forget about the feelings of others.)

Ask the children, "What do you think that Tom was feeling when Jack wouldn't share with him?" (Try to bring out both the notion of feeling hurt, sad, or rejected as well as possibly feeling angry.)

Ask the children, "What could Tom do to help or esteem himself?"

Share with the class that there are no simple answers to this one and that none of the choices Tom has available to him might be completely satisfying . . . but what could he do, anyway?

Have the children color the *I Can Learn to Share* picture (Figure 6.12).

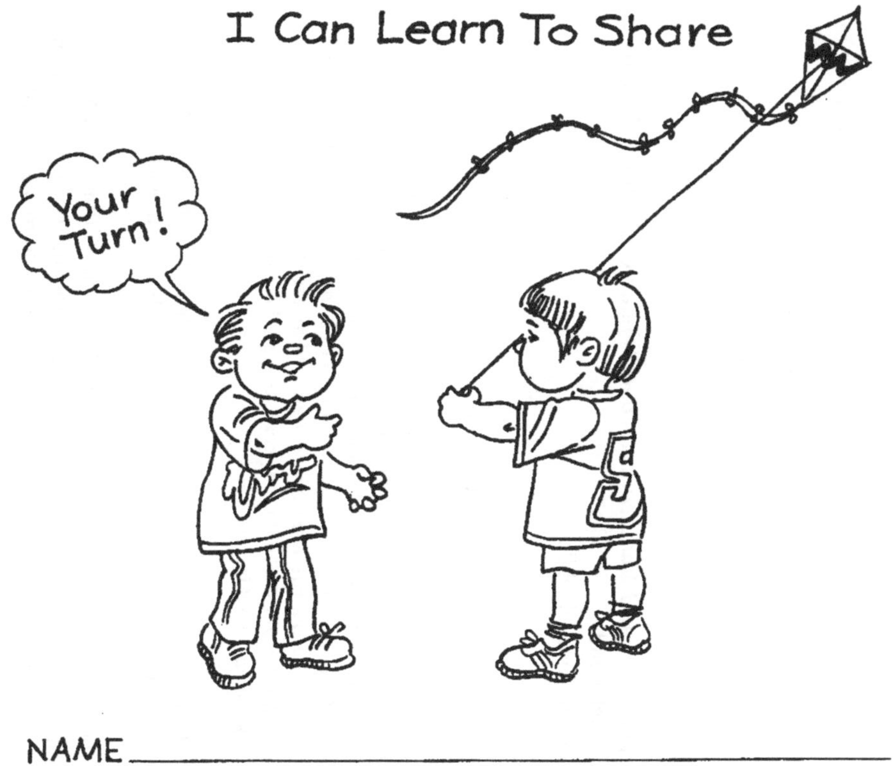

Figure 6.12. I Can Learn to Share. Permission is granted to enlarge and photocopy for classroom use.

ESTEEM EXERCISE 1
(Ages 8 Through 11)

Objective

To help children understand the meaning of esteem and ways to respect and care for themselves and others simultaneously.

Activity

Tell the children that Grandpa Jim is coming back to tell them more about mental muscles. Tell them that you want to read them another story about Grandpa Jim because he is going to give them some more information about another mental muscle called esteem.

Tell the children that you want them to listen carefully because you will ask them to tell you what happened in the story.

Read the Esteem Vignette to the children located at the beginning of the Esteem section. Now, with each section of the vignette, ask the children to recall what happened next.

Ask the children, "What do you think it means to have esteem or to esteem yourself and others?"

After the children have given you their ideas, tell them that esteem means "that you treat yourself and others like valuable persons, with kindness and respect."

Tell the children that Grandpa Jim knows how to esteem himself and others. Ask them if they know why. Accept several answers.

Now tell the children that Grandpa Jim learned a lot about esteeming or taking care of himself and respecting others from Grandmother Ruth. Then he practiced what he learned.

Tell the children that in the rest of the exercises on esteem, they will learn more about treating themselves and others kindly, with respect.

ESTEEM EXERCISE 2
(Ages 8 Through 11)

Materials

Provide each child with a photocopy of the *I Am a Special Person* page (Figure 6.13).

Activity

Remind the children how Grandpa Jim said that each person is special in their own way. Tell the children that they are going to learn some ways today that each one of them is special.

Ask the children to fill in the blanks on the "I Am A Special Person" page. Read each one of the statements to the children out loud. Then give them time to finish it.

As time permits, allow the children to share with each other ways that they are special.

If a child is having difficulty with finding an answer to the last statement in Figure 6.13, either

a tell the child something you think is special about him/her, or
b ask the class to volunteer ways they think that child is a special person.

I AM A SPECIAL PERSON

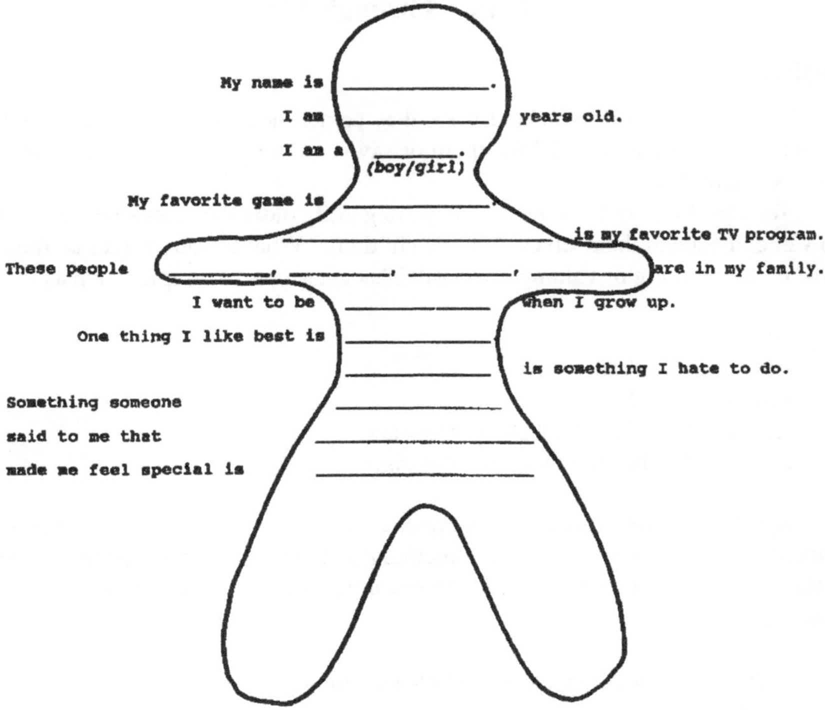

Figure 6.13. I Am a Special Person. Permission is granted to enlarge and photocopy for classroom use.

ESTEEM EXERCISE 3
(Ages 8 Through 11)

Activity

Talk with the children about ways they sometimes feel valuable when other people do something special for them or say something special to them. Accept several examples.

Tell the children that now that they are getting older they can also learn ways to value or esteem themselves. Ask the children, "What actions would be the opposite of esteeming or valuing yourself?" Accept several examples such as

taking drugs,
staying up too late,
eating too much candy,
telling yourself you're a bad person, and
running into the street without looking.

Ask the children to try to remember times in the past when they have said something to themselves or done something that made them feel special or valuable. Some of the following concrete examples may be necessary to begin this discussion.

"I felt good about myself when I cleaned up my room;
brushed my teeth;
looked both ways before I crossed the street;
went to bed on time;
ate foods that were good for me;
said, 'I liked the way I brushed my hair';
shared my candy but didn't give it all away; or
saved some candy for myself."

When the children begin to share their own examples, write their responses on the chalkboard under the heading, "I CAN ESTEEM MYSELF."

With the time remaining, have each child draw a picture of themselves doing something at home or at school that helps them esteem themselves. Display these pictures on a bulletin board titled I CAN ESTEEM MYSELF.

Tell the children that you would like for them to practice esteeming themselves in one of these ways during the next two weeks.

ESTEEM EXERCISE 4
(Ages 8 Through 11)

Activity

Remind the children that last week they discussed ways they could esteem themselves. Take time to let the children discuss how successful they were and ways they could become more successful. Tell them that this week they are going to talk about ways they can esteem each other.

Ask the children to give you several examples of ways that children *don't* value or esteem each other. Accept several examples such as

calling names,
hitting,
picking on someone,
not sharing toys or other things,
leaving someone out, and
always finding what's wrong with another person,

Now, ask the children to try to remember times in the past when they have said or done something that esteemed or valued someone else. Accept several examples such as

sharing,
taking turns,
helping someone with a chore,
giving someone a gift, and
saying something nice about or to someone.

When children begin to share their own examples, write their responses on the chalkboard under the heading, "I CAN ESTEEM OTHERS."

With the time remaining, have each child draw a picture of themselves doing or saying something at home or at school that helps them esteem others. Display these pictures on a bulletin board titled I CAN ESTEEM OTHERS.

Tell the children that you would like them to practice esteeming others in one of these ways during the following week.

ESTEEM EXERCISE 5
(Ages 8 Through 11)

Materials

- Provide each child with a photocopy of the *I Value Myself* page (Figure 6.14).
- Scissors

Activity

Remind the children that last week they discussed ways they could esteem others. Take time to let the children discuss how successful they were and ways they could become more successful in esteeming others.

Tell the children that you want them to look with you at the *I Value Myself* page (Figure 6.14). Read to the children the statements that appear in the box. Ask the children to choose one of the affirmations that are listed below the box and write it in the box, or tell the children they can make up their own.

Ask the children to cut out the box and tape it to their desk as a reminder of one way they are valuable. Tell them to read it to themselves several times a day.

Tell the children that sometimes other people who treat us kindly and esteem us may not receive a thank you for their kindness.

Ask the children to take out a sheet of paper to write a thank you note to someone who has treated them kindly. Provide the following guide on the chalkboard:

> Dear ____________,
>
> Thank you for ______________________________.
>
> What you did helped me feel special.
>
> Sincerely,
>
> Child's Name

Encourage the children to deliver or mail the letter to this person.

I VALUE MYSELF

My name is ______________________________________.

One thing I want to remember this week is

____

____

____

I am special.

I am learning to take care of myself.

I can make mistakes and learn.

I can love me just the way I am.

I don't have to be good at everything.

I am a valuable person.

Figure 6.14. I Value Myself. Permission is granted to enlarge and photocopy for classroom use.

PRACTICAL EXERCISES FOR WISDOM

Vignette (To Be Read with Wisdom Exercise 1)

One day when Tom and Jeri were playing marbles in Jeri's backyard, they noticed that Cody had come outside and was standing on the edge of the back porch. Before they could get to him, Cody went tumbling down the three stairs on the back porch and landed on his hands and knees in the yard. Cody's knees were scratched and bleeding from the fall.

Grandpa Jim was sitting under a tree on the other side of the yard. He came over, picked up Cody, and took him into the house. Tom said, "I hope he's not hurt too bad." Jeri said, "Oh, he'll be all right, but he needs to have his cuts washed and bandaged."

Grandpa Jim came back out in a few minutes and said that Cody was okay, but a little bruised. He said, "Cody was too little to know it was wrong for him to come out on the back porch by himself. He also didn't know what might happen to him if he fell off the porch. He didn't know to be afraid of it. He's got some learning to do."

Grandpa Jim continued, "Remember when we talked about wisdom? It is a mental muscle you need to develop to take care of yourself and get along with other people?" Tom and Jeri nodded.

Grandpa Jim said, "When Cody has more wisdom, he will know more about right and wrong and that it was wrong to do something that was against the rules. He'll think better, too. He'll know that standing on the edge of a porch could make him fall. He'll also learn to be frightened because standing on the edge is dangerous. As Cody grows older, he'll be developing stronger mental muscles. He will know how to think better, how to use his feelings, and how to tell the difference between right and wrong. He will become wiser."

Working Definitions

Wisdom is using your thoughts, feelings, and values to know what is true. Wisdom means using good judgment and acting in a smart way.

Feelings are changes that we experience inside us when things happen to us. They are like an energy system to help us adjust to changes in our lives. If we know what they are, they can help us by giving us energy to cope.

Thoughts are ideas generated by our brains. We use our thoughts to help us reason, think about what we have done, plan what we will do, and act in a way that makes sense.

Values are what is important to us. We spend time, energy, and sometimes money on things that we value. As children, we learn what to value from adults (e.g., parents, teachers, ministers).

Practice Chart

Make a larger version of the *Wisdom Practice Chart* (Figure 6.15). The chart should be large enough to be seen by children in a classroom setting.

Children need practice and exercise to develop strong mental muscles. The chart will be used as a reminder and reinforcement to the children of times when they are acting wisely.

Look for times during the week when feelings are owned and expressed, when thoughts are used in a helpful way, and/or when someone has acted in a respectful way to self and others.

Put names and incidents on the practice chart. Keep adding to the lists, praising children for expressing feelings, for thinking, and for acting wisely.

WISDOM PRACTICE CHART

I Feel	I Think	I Do the "Right" Thing
(owning and coping with feelings)	(owning and exercising thinking)	(acting in a way that is respectful to oneself and others)
Example: Jim said he felt "angry" but did not hit someone.	Example: Phyllis thought of a way to finish her math problems. (She quit talking to her neighbor.)	Example: Robert and Joanna shared the swing and took turns together.

Figure 6.15. Wisdom Practice Chart.

WISDOM EXERCISE 1
(Ages 5 Through 7)

Objective

To help children understand the meaning of wisdom and how their own thoughts, feelings, and values are growing stronger as they understand and use them.

Activity

Remind the children that Grandpa Jim told Tom and Jeri he would be telling them more about mental muscles. Tell them that you want to read them a story about Grandpa Jim because he is coming back to give them some more information about a mental muscle called wisdom. Tell the children that you want them to listen carefully because you will ask them to tell you what happened in the story.

Read the Wisdom Vignette located at the beginning of the Wisdom section to the children.

Now, with each section of the vignette, ask the children to recall what happened next. Ask the children, "What do you think it means to have wisdom or to be wise?"

After the children have given you their ideas, tell the children that wisdom means "knowing about things, knowing what is true, and knowing the right thing to do. It means using good judgment."

Tell the children that Grandpa Jim is wise. Ask them if they know why. Accept several answers.

Now tell the children that Grandpa Jim is wise because he's learned a lot. He knows a lot about his feelings, he is able to think for himself, and he knows the right thing to do. Tell the children that sometimes Grandpa Jim makes mistakes, too, but that he has learned from his mistakes.

Tell the children that, in the rest of the exercises on wisdom, they will learn more about their feelings, their thoughts, and the right thing to do. They will become a little wiser and will be building their mental muscles.

WISDOM EXERCISES 2, 3, AND 4
(Ages 5 Through 7)

In the next three exercises, please follow the activity procedure shown below. In Exercise 2, focus on feelings; in Exercise 3, on thoughts; and in Exercise 4, on values.

Activity

Ask the children the following questions:

What does it mean tor ____________________?

- have feelings (Exercise 2)
- think (Exercise 3)
- know the difference between right and wrong (Exercise 4)

How do we learn to ____________________?

- know what to feel (Exercise 2)
- know what to think (Exercise 3)
- know the difference between right and wrong (Exercise 4)

How can ____________________ help us develop our mental muscles and become a strong separate person?

- knowing our feelings (Exercises 2)
- thinking (Exercise 3)
- knowing the difference between right and wrong (Exercise 4)

(Accept examples from the children's own lives.)

What happens if we don't ____________________?

- know our feelings (Exercise 2)
- think (Exercise 3)
- know the difference between right and wrong (Exercise 4)

(Accept examples from the children's own lives.)

Tell the children that you will notice and you want *them* to notice times when they ___________________.

- express their feelings (Exercise 2)
- think (Exercise 3)
- know right from wrong (Exercise 4)

Bring to the children's attention and record on the *Wisdom Practice Chart* (Figure 6.15) good examples of expressing feelings (Exercise 2), thinking (Exercise 3), and knowing right from wrong (Exercise 4), reminding them that they are building mental muscles.

Have the children color the appropriate *I Can Build Mental Muscles* picture. Use the *Knowing My Feelings* picture (Figure 6.16) for Exercise 2, the *Thinking* picture (Figure 6.17) for Exercise 3, and the *Knowing Right from Wrong* picture (Figure 6.18) for Exercise 4.

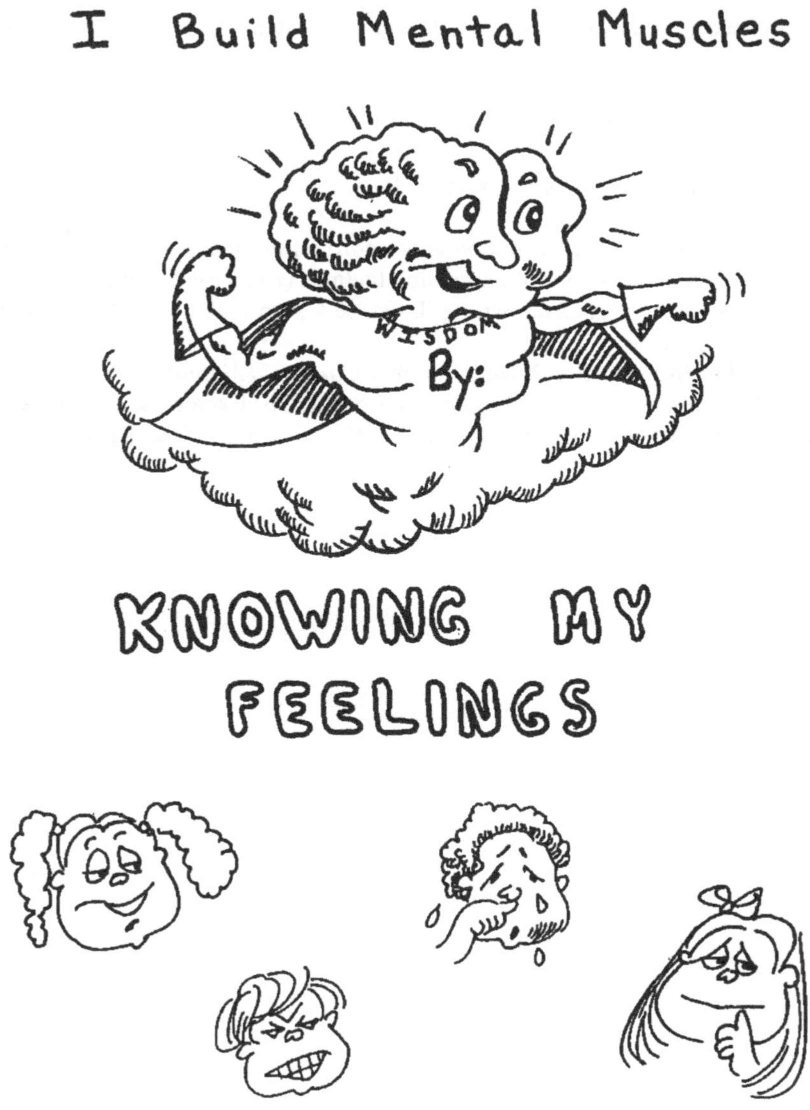

Figure 6.16. I Build Mental Muscles—Knowing My Feelings. Permission is granted to enlarge and photocopy for classroom use.

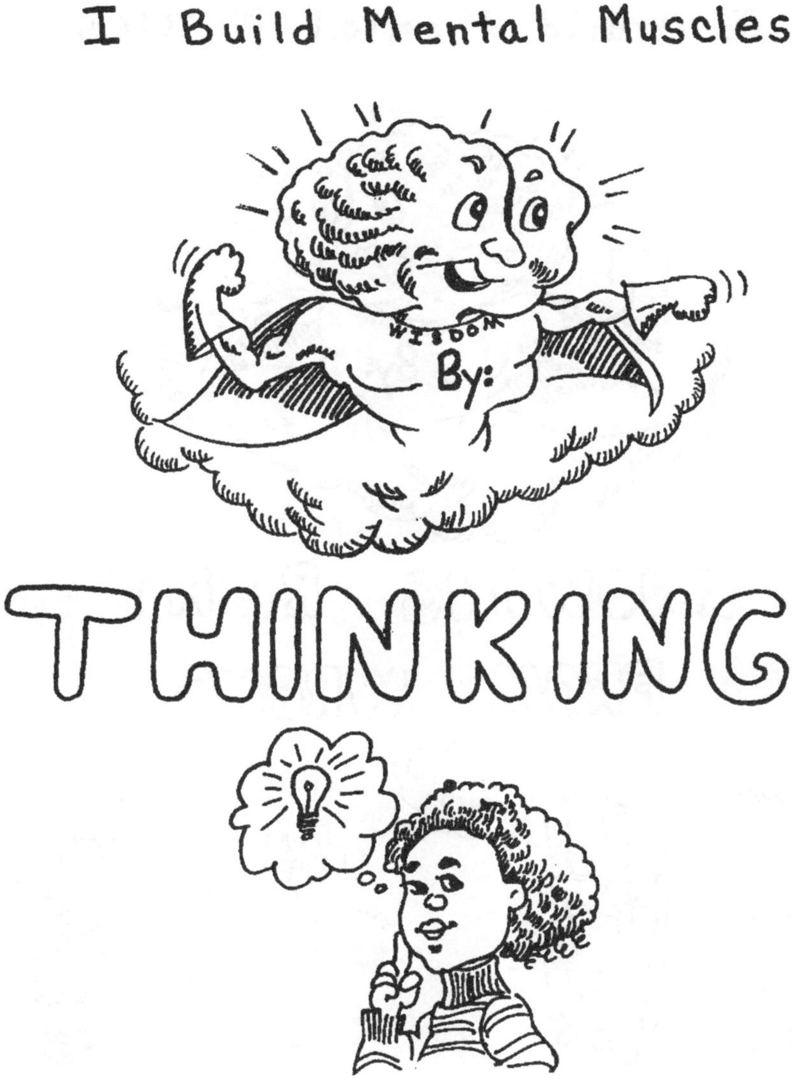

Figure 6.17. I Build Mental Muscles—Thinking. Permission is granted to enlarge and photocopy for classroom use.

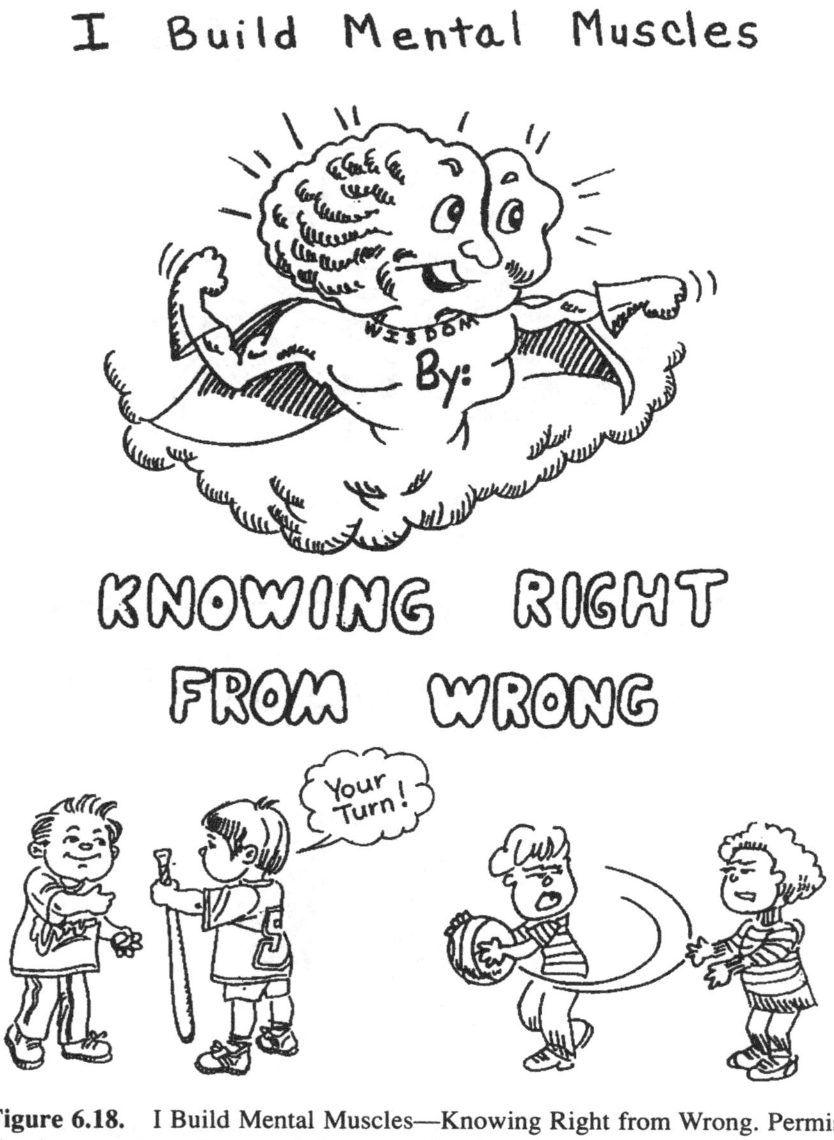

Figure 6.18. I Build Mental Muscles—Knowing Right from Wrong. Permission is granted to enlarge and photocopy for classroom use.

WISDOM EXERCISE 5
(Ages 5 Through 7)

Activity

Reread the Wisdom Vignette to the children. After you have finished, ask the children as a group to take turns telling the vignette again, this time pretending that Cody is their age and that he has built mental muscles.

Tell the children that you want them to tell the story differently because now Cody will know what he is feeling (i.e., he might have fear of falling off step); he will know how to think (i.e., he would know that he'd better not stand on the edge of the step because he might fall); and he would know right from wrong (i.e., maybe he would have told his mother that he was going outside to play).

Have the children talk about how they have grown in wisdom. Then have the children talk about other people who they believe are wise—people who have strong mental muscles and who know and express their feelings, think, and do the right thing. Accept several examples. With each example, have the child say why they think the person is wise.

Have the children say one thing they might work on to be wiser and have stronger mental muscles in the months ahead.

If time remains, have the children draw a picture of themselves doing this activity. Display the pictures on bulletin board under the following titles:

Knowing My Feelings **Thinking** **Doing the Right Thing**

WISDOM EXERCISE 1
(Ages 8 Through 11)

Objective

To help children understand the meaning of wisdom and how their own thoughts, feelings, and values are growing stronger as they understand and use them.

Activity

Remind the children that Grandpa Jim told Tom and Jeri he would be telling them more about mental muscles. Tell them that you want to read them a story about Grandpa Jim because he is coming back to give them some more information about a mental muscle called wisdom. Tell the children that you want them to listen carefully because you will ask them to tell you what happened in the story.

Read the Wisdom Vignette located at the beginning of the Wisdom section to the children.

Now, with each section of the vignette, ask the children to recall what happened next. Ask the children, "What do you think it means to have wisdom or to be wise?"

After the children have given you their ideas, tell the children that wisdom means "knowing about things, knowing what is true, and knowing the right thing to do. It means using good judgment."

Tell the children that Grandpa Jim is wise. Ask them if they know why. Accept several answers.

Now tell the children that Grandpa Jim is wise because he's learned a lot. He knows a lot about his feelings, he is able to think for himself, and he knows the right thing to do. Tell the children that sometimes Grandpa Jim makes mistakes, too, but that he has learned from his mistakes.

Tell the children that, in the rest of the exercises on wisdom, they will learn more about their feelings, their thoughts, and the right thing to do. They will become a little wiser and will be building their mental muscles.

WISDOM EXERCISES 2, 3, AND 4
(Ages 8 Through 11)

Materials

Provide each child a copy of *My Wisdom Journal* (Figure 6.19).

Activity

Review the working definitions of wisdom, feelings, thoughts, and values.

Ask the children to read along silently while you read aloud one page of Figure 6.19 (Journal Day 1 for Exercise 2, Journal Day 2 for Exercise 3, or Journal Day 3 for Exercise 4) of *My Wisdom Journal*.

Give the children time each day to complete the activity (15 minutes), and leave 15 minutes for discussion and sharing.

MY WISDOM JOURNAL

DAY 1

Think of someone you know who you think is wise and has strong mental muscles. Write this person's name below and/or draw a picture of this person.

Name: ______________________________

Picture:

Why is this person wise?

Think of a time when you believe you acted wisely, when you were using you mental muscles. Write and/or draw a picture about the time you were wise.

Picture:

Think of a time when you believe you did *not* act wisely. Write and/or draw a picture below about it.

Picture:

Figure 6.19. My Wisdom Journal, Day 1. Permission is granted to enlarge and photocopy for classroom use.

MY WISDOM JOURNAL

DAY 2

In the next week, choose a time or situation when you might need to act wisely. Write or draw below about that situation.

Picture:

What would be a wise thing to do in that situation? Write or draw below.

Picture:

Why is this wise? Write or draw below.

Picture:

Figure 6.19., Continued. My Wisdom Journal, Day 2. Permission is granted to enlarge and photocopy for classroom use.

MY WISDOM JOURNAL

DAY 3

Wisdom means using your thoughts, feelings, and values to know what is true. It means using good judgment and acting in a "smart way."

Think of a time last week when you needed to use your thoughts, feelings, or values to help you act in a "smart way." Describe and/or draw the situation below.

Picture:

Describe and/or draw whether you used or did not use wisdom on this day. Include whether or not you used your thoughts, feelings, or values.

Picture:

Write and/or draw below why this was wise or not wise.

Picture:

Figure 6.19., Continued. My Wisdom Journal, Day 3. Permission is granted to enlarge and photocopy for classroom use.

WISDOM EXERCISE 5
(Ages 8 Through 11)

Activity

Divide the children into groups of 6.

Tell the children that you want them to come up with a situation that happens in school where children need to be wise, using thoughts, feelings, and values to know what is true and to act in a "smart way."

Ask the children to think of a way to act out (role-play) their situation for the rest of the class. Each person needs to have a role in the role-play. Tell the children to role-play their situation once with a non-wise ending. Then tell them you want them to role-play it a second time with a wise ending.

Have the group and the rest of the class discuss why they think one ending was not wise and the other was wise.

Can anyone in the class tell whether thoughts, feelings, and values were used wisely? How?

REFERENCES

Allen, S., & Dlugokinski, E. (1992). *I am special*. Raleigh, NC: Feelings Factory.

Altshuler, J. L., & Ruble, D. N. (1989). Developmental changes in children's awareness of strategies for coping with uncontrollable stress. *Child Development, 60,* 1337–1349.

Amato, P. R., & Keith, B. (1991). Parental divorce and the well-being of children: A meta-analysis. *Psychological Bulletin, 110*(1), 26–46.

Ankenbrandt, M. J. (1986). Learned resourcefulness and other cognitive variables related to divorce adjustment in children. *Dissertation Abstracts International, 47,* 5045B - 4046B, DA 8628750.

Arendell, T. (1995). *Fathers and divorce*. Thousand Oaks, CA: Sage Publications.

Attar, B. K., Guerra, N. G., & Tolan, P. H. (1994). Neighborhood disadvantage, stressful life events, and adjustment in urban elementary-school children. *Journal of Clinical Child Psychology, 23,* 391–400.

Band, E. B., & Weisz, J. R. (1988). How to feel better when it feels bad: Children's perspectives on coping with everyday stress. *Developmental Psychology, 24,* 247–253.

Bandura, A. (1977). Self-efficacy: Toward a unifying theory of behavioral change. *Psychological Review, 84,* 191–215.

Bellingham, R., Cohen, B., Jones, T., & Spanoil, L. (1989, October). Connectedness. *American Journal of Health Promotion*.

Bevelle, S. L., & Nickerson, C. (1981). *Improving the quality of work: A strategy for delinquency prevention*. Washington, DC: Department of Justice.

Blatt, S. J., & Shichman, S. (1983). Two primary configurations of psychopathology. *Psychoanalysis and Contemporary Thought, 6,* 187–254.

Blos, P. (1979). *The adolescent passage.* New York: International Universities Press.

Brown, J. H., Eichenberger, S. A., Portes, P. R., & Christensen, D. N. (1992). Family functioning factors associated with the adjustment of children of divorce. *Journal of Divorce & Remarriage, 17*(1/2), 81–95.

Browne, A., & Finkelhor, D. (1986). Impact of child sexual abuse: A review of the research. *Psychological Bulletin, 99,* 66–77.

Burbach, D. J., & Peterson, L. (1986). Children's concepts of physical illness: A review and critique of the cognitive developmental literature. *Health Psychology, 5,* 307–325.

California Task Force to Promote Self-Esteem and Social Responsibility. (1990). *Toward a state of esteem: A final report.* Sacramento, CA: California State Department of Education.

Camara, K. A., & Resnick, G. (1989). Styles of conflict resolution and cooperation between divorced parents: Effects on child behavior and adjustment. *American Journal of Orthopsychiatry, 59*(4), 560–573.

Caplan, G. (1980). An approach to preventive intervention in child psychiatry. *Canadian Journal of Psychiatry, 25,* 671–682.

Compas, B. E. (1987). Coping with stress during childhood and adolescence. *Psychological Bulletin, 101,* 393–403.

Compas, B. E., Banez, G. A., Malcarne, V., & Worsham, N. (1991). Perceived control and coping with stress: A developmental perspective. *Journal of Social Issues, 47*(4), 23–34.

Consortium on the School-Based Promotion of Social Competence. (1991). Preparing students for the twenty-first century: Contributions of the prevention and social competence promotion fields. *Teacher College Record, 93,* 297–305.

Coopersmith, S. (1967). *The antecedents of self-esteem.* San Francisco: W. H. Freeman.

Cowen, E. L., Hightower, A. D., Pedro-Carroll, J., & Work, W. (1990). School-based models for primary prevention programming with children. In R. P. Lorion

(Ed.), *Protecting the children: Strategies for optimizing emotional and behavioral development* (pp. 133–160). New York: Haworth.

Crouch, J. L., & Milner, J. S. (1993). Effects of child neglect on children. *Criminal Justice and Behavior, 20,* 49–65.

Custer, G. (1994, October). Balance can counteract stress of work. *APA Monitor,* 49–50.

Denham, S. A., & Almeida, M. C. (1987). Children's social problem-solving skills, behavioral adjustment and interventions: A meta-analysis evaluation of theory and practice. *Journal of Applied Developmental Psychology, 8,* 391–409.

Dlugokinski, E. (1987). *Coping.* Raleigh, NC: Feelings Factory.

Dlugokinski, E. (1990). *Caring connections without co-dependency.* Raleigh, NC: Feelings Factory.

Dlugokinski, E., & Allen, S. (1991). *Caring connections.* Raleigh, NC: Feelings Factory.

Dlugokinski, E., & Allen, S. (1994a). *Living in self esteem.* Raleigh, NC: Feelings Factory.

Dlugokinski, E., & Allen, S. (1994b). *The secret of work and play.* Raleigh, NC: Feelings Factory.

Dlugokinski, E., Allen, S., Russner, W., Collins, T., & Fischer, P. (1994, August). *Prevention strategies in elementary school settings.* Symposium presented at American Psychological Association convention, Los Angeles, CA.

Dlugokinski, E., & Suh, H. (1989). *Enhancing emotional competence: A handbook of exercises for teachers and therapists.* Raleigh, NC: Feelings Factory.

Drotar, D. (1994). Impact of parental health problems on children: Concepts, methods, and unanswered questions. *Journal of Pediatric Psychology, 19,* 525–536.

Dryfoos, J. G. (1990). *Adolescents at risk: Prevalence and prevention.* New York: Oxford University Press.

Dubow, E. F., Schmidt, D., McBride, J., Edwards, S., & Merk, F. L. (1993). Teaching children to cope with stressful experiences: Initial implementation and evaluation of a primary prevention program. *Journal of Clinical Child Psychology, 22*(4), 428–440.

Eiser, C., & Eiser, J. R. (1987). Explaining illness to children. *Communication and Cognition, 20*, 277–290.

Elkind, D. (1981). *The hurried child: Growing up too fast too soon.* Massachusetts: Addeson- Welsey Publishing.

Erikson, E. (1968). *Identity: Youth and crisis.* New York: W.W. Norton.

Finkelhor, D., & Dziuba-Leatherman, J. (1994). Victimization of children. *American Psychologist, 49*(3), 173–183.

Forehand, R., Thomas, A. M., Wierson, M., Brody, G., & Fauber, R. (1990). Role of maternal functioning and parenting skills in adolescent functioning following parental divorce. *Journal of Abnormal Psychology, 99*, 278–283.

Fosson, A., Martin, J., & Haley, J. (1990). Anxiety among hospitalized latency-age children. *Developmental and Behavioral Pediatrics, 11*, 324–328.

Gallo, A. M., Breitmayer, B. J., Knafl, K. A., & Zoeller, L. H. (1992). Well siblings of children with chronic illness: Parents' reports of their psychological adjustment. *Pediatric Nursing, 18*(1), 23–27.

Garbarino, J., Dubrow, N., Kostelny, K., & Pardo, C. (1992). *Children in danger: Coping with the consequences of community violence.* San Francisco: Jossey-Bass.

Garbarino, J., Kostelny, K., & Dubrow, N. (1991). *No place to be a child: Growing up in a war zone.* Lexington, MA: Lexington Books.

Gately, D. W., & Schwebel, A. I. (1991). The challenge model of children's adjustment to parental divorce explaining post-divorce outcomes in children. *Journal of Family Psychology, 5*(1), 60–81.

Glass, D. D. (1985). Onset disability in a parent: Impact on child and family. In S. K. Thurman (Ed.), *Children of handicapped parents: Research and clinical perspectives* (pp. 145–154). Orlando, FL: Academic Press.

Glenn, S. H., & Nelson, J. (1988). *Raising self-reliant children in a self-indulgent world.* Rocklin, CA: Prima Publishing and Communications.

Guidubaldi, J., Cleminshaw, H. K., Perry, J., Nastasi, B. K., & Lightel, J. (1986). The role of selected family environment factors in children's post-divorce adjustment. *Family Relations, 35,* 141–151.

Guisinger, S., & Blatt, S. J. (1994). Individuality and relatedness. *American Psychologist, 49*(2), 104–111.

Hackett, L. (1993). Normal development and specific developmental delays. In D. Black & D. Cottrell (Eds.), *Seminars in child and adolescent psychiatry* (pp. 6–27). Glasgow: Bell and Bain, Ltd.

Hancock, M., Gager, P., & Elias, M. (1993). *School implementation study and findings from a statewide survey.* A working paper obtained from Rutgers University, Department of Psychology, New Brunswick, NJ.

Hawkins, J., Catalano, R., & Miller, J. (1992). Risk and protective factors for alcohol and other drug problems in adolescence and early adulthood: Implications for substance abuse prevention. *Psychological Bulletin, 112,* 64–105.

James, J. W., & Cherry, F. (1988). *The grief recovery handbook: A step-by-step program for moving beyond loss.* New York: Harper & Row.

Janis, I. (1971). *Stress and frustration.* New York: Harcourt Brace Jovanovich.

Jessor, R. (1991). Risk behavior in adolescence: A psychosocial framework for understanding and action. *Journal of Adolescent Health, 12,* 597–605.

Johnston, M., Martin, D., Martin, M., & Gumaer, J. (1992). Long-term parental illness and children: Perils and promises. *The School Counselor, 39,* 225–231.

Jung, C. (1961). *Memories, dreams, and reflections.* New York: Vintage Books.

Kashani, J. H., Deuser, W., & Reid, J. C. (1991). Aggression and anxiety: A new look at an old notion. *Journal of the American Academy of Child and Adolescent Psychiatry, 30*(2), 218–223.

Kazdin, A. E. (1993). Adolescent mental health. *American Psychologist, 48*(2), 127–141.

Kempe, R. S., & Kempe, C. H. (1978). *Child abuse.* Cambridge: Harvard University Press.

Kerns, D. L., & Rutter, M. L. (1991, September). *Data analysis of the medical evaluation of 1,000 suspected sexual abuse victims*. Paper presented at the Ninth Annual Conference on Child Abuse & Neglect, Denver, CO.

Koeppen, A. (1974, October). Relaxation training for children. *Elementary School Guidance and Counseling*, 14–21.

Kohlberg, L. (1984). *Essays on moral development: Vol. II. The psychology of moral development*. New York: Harper and Row.

Kohut, H. (1971). *The analysis of the self*. New York: International Universities Press.

Koocher, G. P., & Gudas, L. J. (1992). Grief and loss in childhood. In C. E. Walker & M. C. Roberts (Eds.), *Handbook of clinical child psychology* (pp. 1025–1034). New York: John Wiley & Sons.

Lazarus, R. S., & Folkman, S. (1984). *Stress, appraisal and coping*. New York: Springer.

Lewis, R., Dlugokinski, E., Caputo, L., & Griffin, R. (1988). Children at risk: Risk and resource dimensions. *Clinical Psychology Review, 8*, 417–440.

Lore, R. K., & Schultz, L. A. (1993). Control of human aggression. *American Psychologist, 48*(1), 16–25.

Lykken, D. T. (1993). Predicting violence in the violent society. *Applied and Preventive Psychology, 2*(1), 13–20.

McEvoy, A. (1994). In C. Turkington (Ed.), Youth gangs: Symptom of nations social woes. *APA Monitor, 25*(2), 32–33.

Mahler, M. S. (1968). *On human symbiosis and the vicissitudes of individuation*. New York: International Universities Press.

Martin, T. C. & Bumpus, L. L. (1989). Recent trends in marital disruption. *Demography, 26*(1), 37–51.

Michelson, L. (1987). Cognitive-behavioral strategies in the prevention and treatment of antisocial disorders in children and adolescents. In J. Burchard & S. Burchard (Eds.), *Prevention of delinquent behavior* (pp. 275–310). Newbury Park, CA: Sage.

Morehead, P. (1991). *The new American Roget's college thesaurus*. New York: Signet Books.

Moshman, D., Glover, J., & Bruning, R. (1987). *Developmental psychology*. Boston: Little, Brown, & Co.

Nicholson, A. C., Titler, M., Montgomery, L. A., Kleiber, C., Craft, M. J., Halm, M., Buckwalter, K., & Johnson, S. (1993). Effects of child visitation in adult critical care units: A pilot study. *Heart & Lung, 22,* 36–45.

Nolen-Heoksema, S. (1992). Children coping with uncontrollable stressors. *Applied and Preventive Psychology, 1*(4), 183–189.

Olson, D. H., Russell, C. S., & Sprenkle, D. H. (1983). Circumplex model of marital and family systems: IV. Theoretical update. *Family Process, 22,* 69–83.

Pavlov, I. P. (1927). *Conditioned reflexes*. London: Oxford University Press.

Pedro-Carroll, J. L., & Cowen, E. L. (1985). The children of divorce intervention program: An investigation of the efficacy of a school based prevention program. *Journal of Consulting and Clinical Psychology, 53,* 603–611.

Peterson, L. (1989). Coping by children undergoing stressful medical procedures: Some conceptual, methodological, and therapeutic issues. *Journal of Consulting and Clinical Psychology, 57,* 380–387.

Peterson, J. L., & Zill, N. (1986). Marital disruption, parent-child relationships, and behavior problems in children. *Journal of Marriage and the Family, 48,* 295–307.

Peterson, L., & Shigetomi, C. (1981). The use of coping techniques to minimize anxiety in hospitalized children. *Behavior Therapy, 12*(1), 1–14.

Piaget, J. (1963). *The origins of intelligence in children*. New York: Norton. (Original work published 1936)

Pransky, J. (1991). *Prevention—the critical need*. Springfield, MO: The Burrell Foundation.

Prinz, R. J., Blechman, E. A., & Dumas, J. E. (1994). An evaluation of peer coping skills training for childhood aggression. *Journal of Clinical Child Psychology, 23,* 193–203.

Roberts, M. (1988, February). School yard menace. *Psychology Today,* 54–56.

Roseby, V., & Deutsch, R. (1985). Children of separation and divorce: Effects of a social role-taking group intervention on fourth and fifth graders. *Journal of Clinical Child Psychology, 14*(1), 55–60.

Russner, W. E., Allen, S., Collins, T., & Dlugokinski, E. (1994, April 14). *Enhancing emotional competence in elementary school children.* Paper presented at the Southwestern Psychological Association Conference, Tulsa, OK.

Rutter, M. (1979). Protective factors in children's responses to stress and disadvantage. In M. W. Kent & J. E. Rolf (Eds.), *Primary prevention of psychopathology: Vol. 1. Social competence in children* (pp. 49–74). Hanover, NH: University Press of New England.

Ryan, R., & Lynch, J. (1989). Emotional autonomy versus detachment: Revisiting the vicissitudes of adolescence and young adulthood. *Child Development, 59,* 349–356.

Savitsky, J., & Eby, T. (1979). Emotion awareness and anti-social behavior. In C. Izard (Ed.), *Emotions in personality and psychopathology* (pp. 475–494). New York: Plenum Press.

Schaps, E., et al. (1978). *Primary prevention evaluation research: A review of 127 program evaluations.* Walnut Creek, CA: Pacific Institute for Research and Evaluation.

Schultheis, K., Peterson, L., & Selby, V. (1987). Preparation for stressful medical procedures and person x treatment interactions. *Clinical Psychology Review, 7,* 329–352.

Scott, K. D. (1992). Childhood sexual abuse: Impact on a community's mental health status. *Child Abuse & Neglect, 16,* 285–295.

Sedlak, A. J. (1991). *Supplementary analyses of data on the national incidence of child abuse and neglect.* Rockville, MD: Westat.

Shaw, D. S. (1991). The effects of divorce on children's adjustment: Review and implications. *Behavior Modification, 15*(4), 456–485.

Shure, M. B., & Spivack, G. (1982). Interpersonal problem-solving in young children: A cognitive approach to prevention. *American Journal of Community Psychology, 10,* 341–356.

Siegel, L. J., & Hudson, B. O. (1992). Hospitalization and medical care of children. In C. E. Walker & M. C. Roberts (Eds.), *Handbook of clinical child psychology* (pp. 845–858). New York: John Wiley & Sons.

Skinner, B. F. (1938). *The behaviors of organisms: An experimental analysis.* New York: Appleton Century Crofts.

Slaby, R. G. (1994). In S. Sardella (Ed.), Prevention is advocated at youth violence briefing. *APA Monitor, 25*(2), 36–37.

Sleek, S. (1994). Could Prozac replace demand for therapy? *APA Monitor, 25*(4).

Sowder, B. J., Burt, M. R., Rosenstein, M. J., & Milazzo-Sayre, L. J. (1980). *Utilization of psychiatric facilities by children and youth.* Bethesda, MD: Burt Associates.

Stolberg, A. L., & Garrison, K. M. (1985). Evaluating a primary prevention program for children of divorce. *Journal of Clinical Child Psychology, 14,* 49–54.

Stolberg, A. L., & Mahler, J. (1994). Enhancing treatment gains in a school-based intervention for children of divorce through skills training, parental involvement, and transfer procedures. *Journal of Consulting and Clinical Psychology, 62*(1), 147–156.

Titler, M. G., Cohen M. Z., & Craft, M. J. (1991). Impact of adult critical care hospitalization: Perceptions of patients, spouses, children, and nurses. *Heart & Lung, 20,* 174–182.

Urbanska, W. (1991, March). Self-esteem: The hope of the future. *New Woman,* 52–58.

Wall, J. E., & Holden, E. W. (1994). Aggressive, assertive, and submissive behaviors in disadvantaged, inner-city preschool children. *Journal of Clinical Child Psychology, 23,* 382–390.

Wallerstein, J. S. (1983a). Children of divorce: Stress and developmental tasks. In N. Garmezy & M. Rutter (Eds.), *Stress coping and development in children,* (pp. 265–302). New York: McGraw-Hill.

Wallerstein, J. S. (1983b). Children of divorce: The psychological tasks of the child. *American Journal of Orthopsychiatry, 53,* 230–243.

Wallerstein, J. S., & Kelly J. B. (1980). *Surviving the break-up: How children and parents cope with divorce*. New York: Basic Books.

Webster's 21st Century Dictionary. (1993). Nashville, TN: Thomas Nelson.

Weissburg, R. P., Caplan, M. Z., & Sivo, P. J. (1989). A new conceptual framework for establishing school-based social competence programs. In L. A. Bond & B. E. Compas (Eds.), *Primary prevention and promotion in the schools* (pp. 255–296). Newbury Park, CA: Sage.

Weissberg, R. P., & Elias, M. J. (1993). Enhancing young people's social competence and health behavior: An important challenge for educators, scientists, policy-makers, and funders. *Applied and Preventive Psychology, 2,* 179–190.

Wertlieb, D., Weigel, C., & Feldstein, M. (1987). Measuring children's coping. *American Journal of Orthopsychiatry, 57*(4), 548–560.

Wilson-Brewer, R., Cohen, S., O'Donnell, L., & Goodman, I. (1991). *Violence prevention for young adolescents: A survey of the state of the art.* Working paper for the conference, "Violence prevention for young adolescents," Washington, DC, July 1990, Carnegie Corporation.

Wolfe, D. A. (1987). A developmental perspective of the abused child. *Child abuse: Implications for child development and psychopathology.* Newbury Park: Sage Publications.

INDEX

ABOUT THE AUTHORS

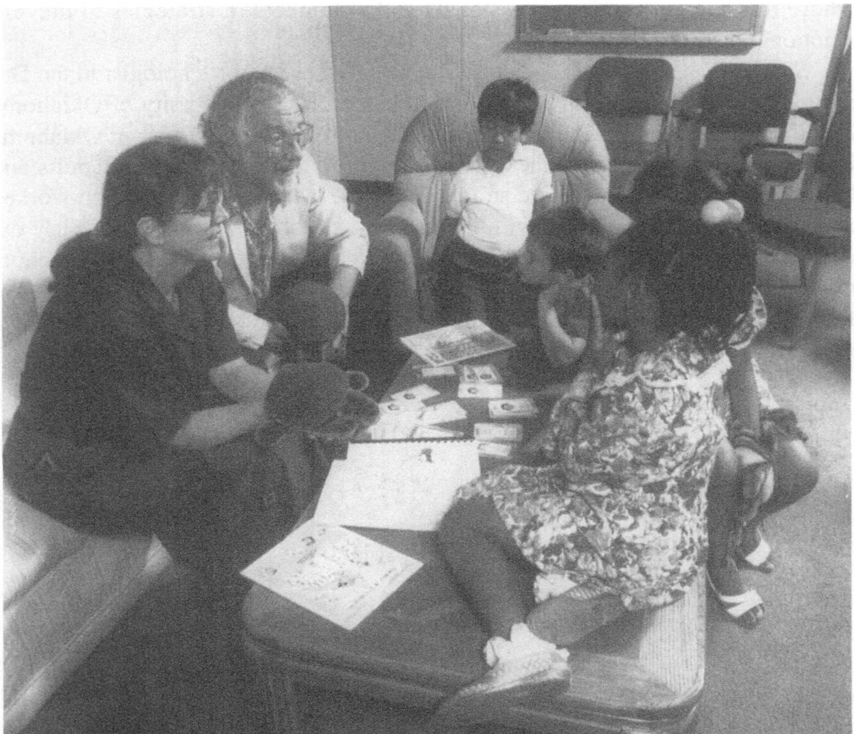

Eric L. Dlugokinski, Ph.D., is a professor in the Department of Psychiatry and Behavioral Sciences at the University of Oklahoma Health Sciences Center. He is coordinator of the Prevention Section in the Department. He began his professional career as a street worker in the City of Detroit and has received awards and honors for distinguished service from several local and national groups. Those include chairing a federal "High Risk Youth" grant review committee and receiving an award from the Oklahoma Psychological Association for Distinguished Contribution to the Public Interest. He received his Ph.D. from Wayne State University in Detroit, MI. Dr. Dlugokinski is a licensed psychologist and has worked in treatment and prevention of emotional disorders for 25 years. He has authored several books and serves as a consultant and grant reviewer in prevention issues. Dr. Dlugokinski is co-director of the Emotional Health Center whose mission is to train professionals and volunteers in strategies to prevent emotional disorders.

Sandra F. Allen, Ph.D., is an assistant professor and psychologist in the Department of Psychiatry and Behavioral Sciences at the University of Oklahoma Health Sciences Center. She received her Ph.D. from the University of Oklahoma in Norman. She works as a therapist with children, adolescents, and adults and has actively pursued preventive strategies for the last 10 years. Dr. Allen worked as a teacher for several years with elementary school children, and her early experience has brought her sensitivity and understanding for teachers and school counselors. She is co-director of the Emotional Health Center and has co-authored several adult and child mental health education curricula with Dr. Dlugokinski.

For Product Safety Concerns and Information please contact our
EU representative GPSR@taylorandfrancis.com Taylor & Francis
Verlag GmbH, Kaufingerstraße 24, 80331 München, Germany